SEVEN WONDERS OF MENOPAUSE

THE MOTHER OF ALL WAKE-UP CALLS

Shavita Kotak

Putting Words
publishing

A catalogue record for this book is available
from the National Library of Australia.

ISBN: 978-1-7637042-2-0 (Paperback)
978-1-7637042-4-4 (Signature Edition – Paperback)
978-1-7637042-3-7 (E-book)

Produced by **Putting Words**
Cover Design by Ashish Joshi
Edited by Eila Jameson-Avey
Proofread by Dave Dennis

Putting Words
PO Box 5062
Wonga Park,
Victoria, 3115
Australia.

www.puttingwords.com
books@puttingwords.com

Contents

"There is no greater power
in the world

than the zest of a
postmenopausal woman."

Margaret Mead

Dedication

This book is lovingly dedicated to Dr. Gladys McGarey, a pioneer, healer, and light whose wisdom and work have shaped the lives of so many, including my own. Dr. McGarey paved the way for a world where healing embraces the whole person—mind, body, and spirit—and reminded us of the importance of listening to our inner knowing.

Her transition to the other side on September 28th, 2024, just days before I was scheduled to meet her, fills me with both deep loss and gratitude. Though I didn't have the chance to sit with her in person, her influence flows through the pages of this book and in the lives of countless others she touched. Her teachings and example leave a legacy that inspires us to seek truth, embrace healing, and create a better world.

This book is also a tribute to the countless women like Dr. McGarey—those who came before us, often at great personal cost, to pave the way for holistic healing. At another time, many of us — myself included—would have been condemned as witches for following our intuition, healing, and sharing ancestral wisdom. Yet these women persisted —speaking, healing, and leading even when it was dangerous to do so. They left footprints so that others, like us, could follow.

Though challenges remain, we carry the light they entrusted to us. This book is not just a tribute, but a continuation of the journey they started—a token of gratitude for all the known and unknown women who came before us and continue to walk with us.

Thank you, Dr McGarey. I see you, hear you, and walk in the light you shared. Together, we are creating a world filled with love.

Acknowledgments

Thank you, God, for guiding this work. I also thank the sacred lands and Indigenous people worldwide whose resilience and wisdom continue to teach us and the ancestors—named and unnamed—whose strength I carry forward. I honour your heritage and feel your presence in every step of this journey.

To every one of the remarkable women who shared their wisdom in this book, you are the true wonders. Dr Gladys McGarey, Ibu Robin Lim, Alexandra Pope, Jane Hardwicke Collings, Dr Christiane Northrup, and Dr Vandana Shiva—your insights and courage light the way for women everywhere. Thank you for trusting me and allowing me to bring your voices together in this work. Your faith in this project has been a gift.

To my parents, thank you for giving me life and for having the courage to uproot your own lives to offer me a better one. Your sacrifices, resilience, and unwavering belief have not been in vain. Each step of my journey is a tribute to the dreams you had for me, and I carry your strength with me every day.

To all migrants worldwide who, like my parents, have left their homelands to create new opportunities for their children—you are the brave ones. In your courage to start anew, you plant the seeds of a better future and leave a lasting legacy of hope and possibility.

To my friends who stand by me, lift me up when I am unsure and celebrate with me through every breakthrough, I owe so much of this work to your belief in me. Thank you for listening, for sharing in my dreams and doubts, and for being there through the tears and laughter.

To my family, thank you for your unwavering love, which reminds me of who I am and why I do this. You are my foundation and my greatest cheerleader.

To every person who has appeared in the pages of my life, to those I have leaned on, laughed with, and grown alongside, thank you. Each of you has left a piece of yourself with me, and I am deeply grateful for the ways you have shaped who I am. This book is my tribute to all of you.

I'd like to thank my patient publisher, Andrea Putting, who held my hand, helped me birth this book, and made this process as smooth as possible. I'm so grateful for your support.

And to you, the readers—the seekers of wisdom—who have dared to explore, learn, and grow through the pages of this book. Your openness to growth and renewal is a gift, and I am honoured to share this journey of healing and transformation with you. ***Thank you.***

The Seven Wonders of Menopause

To the women who came before us,
Whose whispers echo through time,
Their wisdom took root deep in the earth,
Guiding us upward in our climb.

They walked through fire, shadow, and stone,
Their voices were silenced, their stories unknown.
But their strength, like seeds, still grows in us,
A legacy of courage, where rebirth must.

For centuries, the wise were burned and feared,
Their truths erased, their power smeared.
Now we rise from embers and flame,
Reclaiming our voices, shedding the shame.

Menopause—a gateway, not the end—
A time to rise, to break and mend.
Each change a spark, each symptom a guide,
Calling us inward, where truths reside.

This book holds stories bold and true,
A glimpse of what every woman can do.
When we face our shadows and dig deep within,
We rise anew, ready to begin.

To the grandmothers, mothers,
the wise ones of old,
Who suffered in silence, fierce and bold—
We honour you now as we take our place,
Leading the world with feminine grace.

Read with heart, let our stories ignite—
We rise together in truth and light.
And with every step, with every breath,
The best is yet to come.

Introduction

Welcome to The Seven Wonders of Menopause

The Mother of all Wake-up Calls

Inside these pages; you'll find the stories of seven remarkable women who are reshaping humanity with their wisdom, insight, and lived experiences. Together, they share nearly 450 years of accumulated knowledge—a web of wisdom woven from lives dedicated to healing, teaching, and guiding others through the cycles of life.

Each woman's story is written in her own unique style and voice, capturing the individuality and essence of her journey. Each chapter reflects the woman behind it, inviting you to hear her words as if she were speaking directly to you.

Here's who you'll meet in these pages:

- **Dr. Gladys McGarey** — At 103 years old, Dr. Gladys has lived through more than a century of change, embodying resilience and insight that only come with time. Her story is one of endurance, perspective, and the power of living with purpose.

- **Ibu Robin Lim** — Known for her work with mothers and babies, Ibu Robin explores the sacred role of the placenta in welcoming new life, inviting us to reconnect with the beginnings of our own journey.

- **Alexandra Pope** — With a deep reverence for the menstrual cycle, Alexandra guides us through the initiation of womanhood, showing us how our cycles shape our identity, power, and connection to ourselves.

- **Jane Hardwicke Collings** — A keeper of ancient wisdom, Jane teaches about the rites of passage that mark our lives, each stage as a transition in the story of who we are.

- **Dr. Christiane Northrup** — The original menopause doctor, Dr. Northrup brings over 30 years of experience, offering practical and spiritual wisdom on navigating menopause with grace, power, and insight.

- **Dr. Vandana Shiva** — An environmental activist and philosopher, Dr. Shiva reminds us that the planet itself is our mother. Her story draws connections between the cycles of women and the cycles of nature, inspiring us to see ourselves as creators and protectors of life.

And then there's you—and me. We are the seekers of wisdom and knowledge, open to hearing new perspectives, willing to explore different ways of living, and curious about how our journeys intertwine with those of the women who have come before us.

This book is here for you to enjoy at your own pace. When you have a quiet moment, settle in with a warm cup of tea and let each story speak to you. These voices are here to meet you where you are, offering a mirror, a mentor, and a friend in every chapter. By the end, you may realise that you, too, are a wonder—a vital part of this story, with wisdom to share and a journey to honour.

So, take your time, start your journey, and let these stories guide you. This is your space to explore, reflect, and perhaps see yourself in a whole new light.

Why I wrote this book

As I approach one year since my last menstrual cycle, I find myself in a time of deep reflection. My life has been filled with many experiences—heartbreak, financial struggles, joyful moments, and big changes. I've moved countries, switched careers, and faced the ups and downs of raising children, all while going through the stages of womanhood. From the wonder of childbirth to the quiet reflection of menopause, each phase has brought important lessons and helped shape who I am today.

This book comes from my desire to step into this new chapter of life with courage and purpose—on my own terms. For so long, society has mapped out a narrow path for women: education, marriage, motherhood, and the pursuit of security. But now, as I embrace menopause, I feel a new kind of freedom, no longer held back by expectations or the need to fulfil roles others have defined for me. This stage is not a winding down but a coming into my full self, and I know I'm not alone in feeling this.

We need to change the idea that menopause signifies loss, sadness and becoming invisible. **This transition isn't an ending; it's the rebirth of the soul.** Every symptom and experience mirrors a contraction, just like in childbirth. These contractions—whether they come as hot flushes, mood swings, or restless nights—are the body's way of shedding old layers and making space for the soul to emerge, renewed and more powerful than ever. Menopause offers us the chance to be born again, stepping into a version of ourselves that is wiser, freer, and more authentic.

This book is not just about my journey—it's also a collection of stories from remarkable women who have inspired me. Together, we explore the challenges and growth that come with midlife, heal from the past, and create new ways forward for ourselves and future generations. This is about self-discovery, breaking old cycles, and building a new path for our daughters and their children.

I want this book to encourage every woman to see menopause as a chance to grow, heal, and feel empowered. With each page, I invite you to join us on this journey—to grow older without feeling old, welcome change as a friend, and discover the endless possibilities when we embrace life with curiosity and joy. Let this book remind you that the wisdom gained during menopause is exactly what the world needs.

The best is truly yet to come. Menopause is not just the end of fertility, it's the beginning of a vibrant new chapter. This chapter is full of meaning, discovery, and strength. As wise women, it's time to take our place, claim our power, and lead the way forward. This is our rebirth—our souls emerging stronger with every contraction of change, ready to live fully and unapologetically.

Understanding Menopause

Menopause is not just a biological event but the beginning of a personal transformation. It marks the end of one chapter and the beginning of a new one—a rebirth of the soul. Just as childbirth brings contractions that signal the arrival of new life, every symptom of menopause mirrors a contraction, preparing us for the emergence of a wiser, freer version of ourselves.

The Biological Basics

To truly understand menopause, we need to begin with the biological story. At the heart of it all are the ovaries—small but mighty organs responsible for releasing eggs and producing key hormones like oestrogen and progesterone. These hormones regulate the menstrual cycle and influence much more than reproduction—they impact emotions, sleep, bone health, and even heart function.

As the ovaries begin to slow down hormone production during perimenopause (the transition before menopause), the body adjusts. Think of this time as a lead-up to the main event—a period of change that can come with irregular periods, hot flushes, and emotional shifts. Perimenopause is unique for every woman, ranging from a few months to several years, offering signs that the body is preparing for a new rhythm.

Menopause is officially reached after 12 consecutive months without a period. It signals the end of the reproductive phase and the start of something new—an opportunity to explore a different kind of power that comes from within. This shift may bring with it noticeable changes: hot flushes, restless nights, mood swings, and changes in energy levels. While these symptoms can be challenging, they are part of the body's way of recalibrating and creating space for growth and renewal.

The Spiritual Journey of Menopause

Menopause is not just a physical process; it is **The Mother of all Wake-Up Calls.** This life stage invites us to shed old identities and beliefs, much like the leaves of autumn trees, making space for new growth. Every wave of heat, every moment of discomfort, can be seen as a contraction—a signal that transformation is underway, preparing us for a rebirth of the soul.

Just as nature moves through seasons, menopause teaches us that life is a series of cycles, each offering its own opportunities for renewal. This stage is a time to reflect on the journey so far, to honour our achievements, and to realign with what truly matters. It calls us to pause, listen to our intuition, and embrace the wisdom that only comes with experience.

In many cultures, menopause is celebrated as a transition into elderhood, when women become keepers of wisdom and guides for their communities. This is not a time to fade into the background but to take center stage as a source of insight, leadership, and healing. Menopause asks us to lead not with force but with presence—to become grounded in who we are and to share our gifts with the world.

Menopause as a Rebirth

Every symptom of menopause offers a message. The hot flushes burn away old energies, leaving behind clarity and strength. Emotional shifts invite us to release unhealed traumas and open ourselves to new ways of being. Just like contractions in childbirth, these experiences might feel intense, but they guide us toward a deeper connection with ourselves. Through the discomfort, a more authentic version of the self is being born—one that no longer seeks external validation but trusts its inner wisdom.

Menopause allows us to rediscover who we are beyond the roles of mother, daughter, partner or professional. It is a time to nurture ourselves, explore new passions, and reconnect with what brings joy and meaning. We are invited to create a life that reflects our soul's desires filled with curiosity, freedom, and purpose.

This transformation is not always easy, but like childbirth, each challenge brings us closer to something beautiful: a new beginning, a rebirth of the soul, and the opportunity to live fully and authentically. The best part? This chapter offers a unique freedom, the freedom to be exactly who we are without any apologies.

CHAPTER 1

Dr. Gladys McGarey

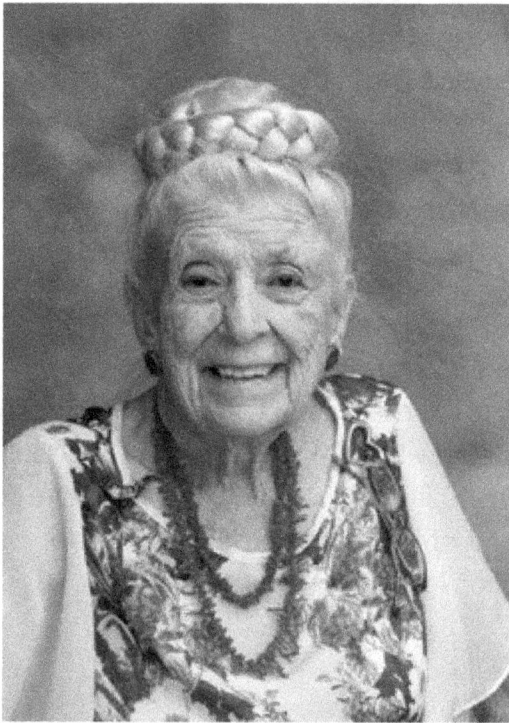

The Fairy Godmother

Introduction to Dr. Gladys McGarey

I first discovered Dr. Gladys McGarey through a series of interviews with Dr. Christiane Northrup, who frequently spoke of her with deep admiration. Intrigued, I began following Dr. McGarey on social media and immersed myself in her many podcast interviews. The connection I felt was immediate—I knew I had to invite her to contribute to this book, and I was incredibly blessed when she accepted.

Learning that she was born in India—a fact that resonated with me as an Indian woman, born in London and now residing in Australia—only heightened my excitement. Dr. McGarey's stories about her time in India, especially her interactions with Gandhi, were fascinating and sparked a deeper connection between us.

I am inspired by Dr. McGarey's spirit and undiminished zest for life despite her many challenges. Her approach to aging and living fully has influenced my own views on aging and menopause. I now see menopause not as an end but as a beginning. If a woman enters menopause in her early 50s and lives into her 80s, she has another 30-plus years ahead—a time filled with growth, change, and renewal.

Reflecting on my past three decades, I see how much I have changed. I've shifted cultures multiple times, moved homes and countries, travelled extensively, experienced love and heartbreak, navigated financial highs and lows, and raised two wonderful children—and now, I'm embarking on writing this book. If the next thirty years are like the past, they will be filled with even more changes and growth. With this perspective, I now welcome menopause, believing that the best is yet to come.

Dr. McGarey's life is rich with history and fills several books. Born in November 1920 to medical missionary parents in India, she became a pioneer in holistic medicine, co-founding the American Holistic Medical Association in 1978.

Throughout her career, she has received numerous medical and lifetime achievement awards. She has authored several impactful books, such as *Born to Live*, *The Physician Within You*, and *Living Medicine*. Her book *The World Needs Old Ladies*, co-authored with Eveline Horelle Dailey, caught my attention while researching for this book. Her latest bestseller, *The Well-Lived Life*, continues to inspire readers around the globe.

In Dr. McGarey, I see not just a medical pioneer but a woman who embodies the potential for growth and wisdom in every stage of life. Her life's work is a testament to the power of embracing each phase of our journey with courage, curiosity, and an open heart.

"Each of us is here to connect
with our unique gifts;

this is what activates our desire
to be alive."

Dr. Gladys McGarey

A Conversation with
Dr. Gladys McGarey

Take a moment to journey back to November 30th, 1920, when I first entered this world, full of energy and excitement. My story began in India, and it started quite dramatically—my mother went into labour with me at the Taj Mahal.

India holds a deep connection to my life. I spent the first 16 years of my childhood there, and I feel incredibly blessed to have grown up in such a unique environment. My parents were medical missionaries working in the jungles of North India, where I spent my early years— travelling in tents, surrounded by the wonders of the jungle.

I remember spending hours playing with the local kids in the jungles. They were fascinated by our differences, often rubbing my arm to see if the 'white' of my skin would come off. Those innocent moments created the foundation of lifelong memories as we explored the wilderness together, growing up side by side.

Attending Woodstock School in the Himalayas was another highlight of my childhood. My sister and I would climb the mountains, especially when the dahlias were in bloom. The vibrant flowers blanketed the landscape, and we'd gather them to bring home, where my mother would lovingly place them all around the house.

Those were special times—filled with beauty, connection, and a deep love for the land and its people. Speaking Hindi and Urdu allowed me to connect deeply with those around me; I understood their world, and they understood mine.

When I was 15, I moved to the States and knew nothing about movie stars. I only knew Princess Margaret and Princess Elizabeth; they were our heroes. So, coming to college in the U.S. was a whole new education. But no matter where life has taken me, growing up in India remains one of the most treasured periods of my life.

I knew I was meant to be a doctor from an early age. Even as a little girl, I would play doctor, treating my dolls for various ailments. My sister wouldn't let me play with her dolls—she didn't want them to get sick! But for me, it was always about helping others get well. I could see myself doing something important, something meaningful, even then.

My mother played a huge role in guiding me; her influence is still with me today. She was an amazing woman. The way she lived her life and helped others was truly inspiring. She passed that on to me, and I've tried to live my life in a way that honours her legacy. It's a living process—what we learn and live, we pass on to others. My mother's way of life was an incredible guide, shaping the path I've chosen to live my life.

Connecting with Mahatma Gandhi

Mahatma Gandhi was very important in my life, especially while I was growing up. He wasn't just a historical figure to me—he was a good friend of my parents, and they worked together during the partition of India. Because of their friendship, Gandhi gave my mother a beautiful cashmere shawl and my father a punny-puck jacket, a type of blanket. It was more than just a professional relationship; it felt like a family connection.

One of my most memorable experiences with Gandhi happened when I was ten. It's something that has stayed with me my entire life. We were on a train returning to the United States. My parents had the opportunity to return home every six and a half years to reconnect with family and friends. This was the first time I would be going to the U.S. that I could remember; honestly, I wasn't happy about it. I loved India and didn't want to leave. I felt so sad, and I remember pressing my face against the train window as we pulled into one of the railway stations.

A big crowd was gathered, but that's typical in India. However, this crowd was different. I noticed a man walking in front, dressed in a dhoti—a simple loincloth—carrying a staff. The people around him were chanting, and I watched, still with my face pressed against the window. Then, something extraordinary happened. Gandhi took a flower from a little girl in the crowd, and as he did, he looked up and gazed directly into my eyes. At that moment, we made a deep connection. Even at the age of ten, I felt a deep soul connection. It isn't easy to put into words. Gandhi understood something about me, and I understood something about him. I've carried this experience with me ever since.

Journey into Medical School

I attended the Woman's Medical College in Philadelphia, the only medical school for women at the time. I started my medical journey in September 1941 and graduated in 1946, which means my entire education took place during the intense backdrop of World War II. It was an incredibly interesting period, with the world undergoing massive changes. I was right in the thick of it, determined to pursue my dream of becoming a doctor.

During my residency, I faced significant challenges. When I started working at a hospital in Cincinnati, Ohio, they had never had a female doctor before and were completely unprepared for my arrival. There were no accommodations for women doctors — no room, no bed — nothing. As a result, there was no place for me to stay when I was on call at night. While the male doctors each had their own room, I had to make do by sleeping on an x-ray table with just a blanket and a pillow. Although it was far from ideal, I didn't complain — I was grateful for the opportunity to practice medicine.

The resident surgeon at that time did not want me to be a woman in medicine. He particularly didn't want me as I was both pregnant and married while in medical school. He believed that pregnant women had no place in the field. He tried everything he could to force me out, but fortunately, he did not succeed. I had dedicated my entire life to achieving this goal, and I wouldn't let anyone who thought they had more power than me force me out. Their desire to see me leave only strengthened my determination to stay.

Journey into Holistic Medicine

I got married in 1943 while I was still in medical school. My husband and I had our first child in 1946; over the years, we were blessed with six children. When I was 35, my family and I relocated to Phoenix, Arizona. By this time, I had connected with a group of physicians who shared my interest in a different approach to medicine. Our education in medical school had focused primarily on disease and its treatment, but we believed there was more to healing than just addressing symptoms. Understanding the patient and the underlying causes of their conditions was crucial to us.

We started communicating and eventually initiated a newsletter to exchange our ideas. As we continued our discussions, it became evident that we needed a more structured organisation to advocate for our comprehensive beliefs, especially since the American Medical Association opposed many of our ideas at the time. We aimed to establish a platform to effectively promote our perspective, whether cooperating with or opposing to existing medical views.

It took us two years to decide on a name because we wanted to emphasise that healing involves the entire being—mind, body, and spirit. We began with the letter 'H' to embody health, healing, and holy concepts. This led to the founding of the American Holistic Medical Association. Initially a small group of like-minded physicians, it has grown significantly and transformed into a prominent integrative health organisation with a powerful presence and influence.

Opening the Olive Tree Medical Group in Phoenix was a natural extension of our efforts. It became a place where we could put our holistic principles into practice, focusing on treating diseases and understanding and caring for the whole person. This journey, from our early ideas to the establishment of a major organisation, has been one of growth and fulfilment, and it continues to shape the way we approach health and healing today.

Edgar Cayce's Influence

When we arrived in Arizona, Edgar Cayce's work impacted us. We bought books that introduced us to his ideas and opened a new area of important thought. His belief that we are spiritual beings living in a physical world aligns perfectly with our approach to medicine. It has become essential to how we practice medicine.

Cayce's approach emphasised that treating patients was about addressing their physical symptoms and engaging with their spiritual aspect. This approach made us feel like we were connecting with something deeper that had always been there.

I remember when my oldest son, Carl, was finishing his medical training. He passed through Phoenix on his way to Del Rio, Texas, and told me, 'Mom, I'm really scared. I'm going out into the world, and I'm going to have people's lives in my hands. I don't know if I can handle that.'

I said to him, 'Carl, if you think you're the one who has the healing power, you have a right to be scared. But if you understand that it's your job to do the orthopaedic work—which is very important—then remember that the healing itself isn't yours. It would be best if you connected with the healer within that patient. The physician within that patient is your colleague. You do your job, and that patient will do their job.'

This idea, inspired by Edgar Cayce's teachings, shaped how we approached medicine. It was about more than the physical; it was about engaging with every part of a person to facilitate healing. This philosophy guided my medical practice and informed the deeper mission of our work in holistic medicine.

Menopause and Aging

This book focuses on menopause, which resonates with me because it emphasises the potential for a vibrant, fulfilling life after this transition. I am 103 years old and am still writing books and sharing my wisdom with the world.

In the 1970s, when I was around 50, menopause was viewed similarly to how it is now. It's a natural part of aging marked by a hormonal shift that every woman goes through. People who had trouble with menopause then, as now, really felt its impact. There wasn't anything wrong with menopause; it was and is about understanding these changes and managing them effectively.

Thankfully, we understand hormonal changes better today than in my medical school days. The key is not to get stuck. Menopause is a natural process—I think of it as **aging into health.** As you transition from adolescence and navigate through the years of raising children, each stage of life requires you to adapt and grow.

If you face hardships and feel stuck, it can be incredibly tough. However, if you view these challenges as opportunities to gain experience and grow, they can become powerful teachers in your life. It's about choosing how you respond and moving forward gracefully and resiliently. When we accept our power, we're the ones who choose.

Be Glad: A Journey to Independence

After 46 years of marriage and all the life we had built together, my husband asked me for a divorce. I was completely blindsided—I had no idea it was coming. The shock was overwhelming, as though the ground beneath me had shifted. My world felt like it was ending, and I was utterly broken.

One day, while driving home from work, the pain became so unbearable that I found myself screaming at the world, at life, in sheer agony. Tears streamed down my face as I struggled to understand it all. Eventually, I had to pull over to the side of the road. I stopped the car, took a deep breath, and stepped out. In that moment of stillness, I thought, 'This is awful. What's happening to me? Are you going to spend the rest of your life feeling this broken, like you can't do anything?' I stood there, truly reflecting on what I was going through and how I was reacting.

Then, out of nowhere, a voice in my head said, **'This is the day the Lord has made. Let us rejoice and be glad in it.'** The word 'glad' struck me deeply as if a ray of hope had pierced through the darkness.

After that moment, a transformation took place within me. When I returned to my empty house, with only my dog there to greet me, I decided to do something. The following day, I replaced the license plate on my car with one that read **'BE GLAD.'** From then on, I drove around

Phoenix with that reminder. Whenever I got into the car, I saw 'BE GLAD.' It served as a declaration of resilience and positivity for me and everyone who noticed it as I drove around town.

Years later, I wrote a letter to my ex-husband, thanking him for giving me my freedom. Before, we were always known as 'Bill and Gladys.' Afterwards, I was simply Gladys, and I had reclaimed my independence. That realisation made me feel truly in charge of my own life.

Life After Divorce

My life after the divorce was nothing short of incredible. I was about 70 years old in 1990, which marked the beginning of a new chapter. Not long after, I travelled to Tibet. My brother, Dr. Carl Taylor, had started an organisation dedicated to global healing. He invited me to join him in Tibet to assist in a workshop aimed at empowering Tibetan women and helping them access their humanity.

At the age of 86, I found myself in Afghanistan, working with Afghan women to improve the birthing process. At that time, Afghanistan had the highest maternal mortality rate in the world, compounded by cultural restrictions that prevented men from speaking to women. My brother invited me to help, giving me a unique opportunity to make a real difference.

Throughout my life, I've been committed to connecting with people and aiding them in their struggles. Reflecting on my past experiences, I realised how different things were. Growing up, I couldn't have imagined even having a telephone, let alone the possibility of communicating with people across the globe. It's a testament to how wonderful and vibrant life is and how our connections with others enrich our lives. It's a wonderful time to be alive.

It's easy to get stuck if you only look for dark spaces. It's like carrying a bag over your shoulder—if you keep looking back at it, your neck will surely get stiff, right? That's why it's crucial to turn your head around and search for the light. If you don't look for it, you won't see it.

The Inspiration Behind The World Needs Old Ladies

As I got older, I entered that stage of life where society tends to label you as an 'old lady.' My friends were in the same place too. One day, a group of remarkable, professional women who had accomplished so much in our fields sat together, and we realised. We looked at each other and said, 'Why don't we claim who we are? The world needs us.'

We had lived rich, full lives, overcome countless challenges, and gathered a wealth of wisdom. Why should we keep all that to ourselves? That's when Evelyn Horrell

Dailey and I decided to write *The World Needs Old Ladies*.

Writing the book was a truly rewarding experience. We explored how to tap into our collective 'inner juice' to enrich our lives and assist others. Our goal was to help people explore dimensions of themselves that they might not have discovered yet. It was about sharing our knowledge and inspiring others to reach new heights and discover new possibilities.

In many traditional cultures, elderly people, especially women, have always played an important role in guiding and developing their communities. It's interesting because many people in our modern society are afraid of getting old. They often talk about aging as something to avoid, always trying to look younger or relive their youth, which I find silly. You've already been young and lived through that time. Now, you have a great opportunity to use your life experiences and share your wisdom with others. This isn't just about getting old; it's about embracing your role as a mentor and guide, using what you've learned to help others find their way.

The Well-Lived Life

Changing how I thought about medicine motivated me to write *The Well-Lived Life*. Before this, all the books I had written were focused on dealing with diseases—they were important and gave me a significant push in my career. However, *The Well-Lived Life* comes from a deeper place. It captures the essence of my experiences working with people and emphasises why I do what I do.

In medical school, I was taught to view medicine as a war against disease and pain. But over time, I realised this wasn't the only way to approach healing. I no longer wanted to see the process as a war to be won against an ailment. Instead, I asked, 'What if these diseases or pains were trying to communicate something to me? What if my body was trying to teach me something through these experiences?' By paying attention to these messages, I learned significant lessons about life.

I wrote *The Well-Lived Life* because it felt necessary after everything I've learned and experienced. The idea came from wanting to capture the essence of living well at every stage of life and finding happiness in every moment. A well-lived life isn't just about reaching goals but also about the wisdom gained along the way. My aim is to share this perspective and offer a guide for treasuring each day.

Life is a Jigsaw Puzzle

I think we all are living examples of how we've lived our lives. It brings me such joy to recognise that my life means something, your life means something, and everybody's life means something. Life is like a vast jigsaw puzzle, and each of us is a unique piece that fits perfectly into a specific place. We're the only ones who can fill that space because it's ours. We've created it, and no one else can fit in that spot.

If we can look at life this way, it transforms our daily steps into something more meaningful. For example, my son John, who helps me with all kinds of things, recently had an experience that illustrates this idea beautifully. He was heading out to his car, and as he went to step in, he noticed a puzzle piece lying in the dirt. It was like it had been waiting for him, and he recognised it as his.

We all have moments like that—puzzle pieces waiting to be recognised and placed. I'm trying to say that we all have that special place in the universe that's uniquely ours. Acknowledging this, we start to see our roles and responsibilities not as burdens but as exhilarating opportunities. It's a huge responsibility, but boy, is it fun. It truly is a privilege to be on this planet.

Connecting with Dreams and Past Lives

Whenever I'm grappling with a question or need to dig deeper into my thoughts and experiences, I make it a point to focus on it before I go to sleep. I'll formulate the question in my mind, and often, when I wake up, I find that I've received an answer—a new perspective that helps me move forward in ways I might not have otherwise considered.

For example, my early struggles with dyslexia. As a child, I had to repeat the first grade because I couldn't read. The letters on the page seemed like a jumble to me.

By the time I reached third grade, I was able to get past the stigma associated with my initial years in school, not because I had mastered reading but because of a teacher named Ms. McGee, who saw something in me that others hadn't. In my first two years of school, I was labelled the class dummy, and the other kids treated me accordingly. However, Ms McGee recognised that, while I couldn't read, I could think critically and articulate my thoughts. She appointed me as the class governor, giving me a role that allowed me to use my strengths.

This experience taught me an important lesson: we don't have to be defined by our limitations. We can move beyond them. However, even as I grew older, became a practising physician, and wrote books, I often found myself questioning my voice. Was I saying the right thing? Was I doing it properly? I'd write something and then ask my husband Bill or someone else to look it over, seeking validation.

I've found that connecting with my dreams and inner guidance has been really important in helping me deal with my doubts and growth. This process keeps shaping my journey.

Trusting My Voice at 93

It wasn't until I was 93 that I truly began to understand and trust my voice, and it all started with a remarkable dream. In this dream, I was my nine-year-old self, emerging from a tent in the jungle where we lived. I was sneaking out, cautiously checking to ensure my younger brother wasn't nearby to tattle on me and get me into trouble. Seeing he wasn't around, I seized the moment, sprinting as fast as I could to a mango tree and climbing all the way to the top.

Perched high in the branches, I began to sing joyously, in the freedom of being where no one could hear me. But then, something surprising happened. I looked over my shoulder and saw Jesus sitting in the tree with me. This scene was so vivid—Jesus, right there, sharing that serene moment with me. I turned to him and said, 'Jesus loves the little children, right?' He laughed warmly and said, 'Yes.' Encouraged, I kept singing, but then I paused, wondering if he really meant it. So, I asked again, 'I'm still one of the little children, right?' And again, he affirmed, 'Yes.'

I resumed singing, and when I awoke from the dream, I was still laughing and singing. That moment struck me deeply—if Jesus thought it was okay, I needed to start accepting my voice. Even at 93, it was clear: what I say is important. I need to listen to my voice and share it with others.

Since that awakening, I've embraced the opportunity to share my wisdom and experiences through my books, various podcasts and social media platforms. Sharing these stories—from the towering mango trees of my youth to the lessons learned along my journey—has been both a privilege and a joy.

The Five L's: A Guide to a Well-Lived Life

The lessons I've taught, especially the Five L's referenced in my book *The Well-Lived Life*, are particularly relevant for women transitioning through menopause. We all encounter opportunities for growth and understanding throughout our lives. If we can recognise these moments as lessons, discover our purpose, and strive to fulfil it, then every aspect of life becomes significant. We begin to see everything as a teacher, and life becomes important in how it's lived.

As we navigate through life, we can either drag ourselves through it or truly live it. When you fully embrace living and understand that love is the ultimate healer, life transforms into something remarkable. I've conceptualised the Five L's in my personal philosophy, which has tremendously helped me navigate this journey.

The first two L's, **Life** and **Love**, are inherently linked. They work together like a pregnancy: whatever I consume, the baby consumes; whatever thoughts I have, the baby experiences. But eventually, the baby emerges as a separate entity, takes its first breath, and transitions from our shared existence to an independent life. This process symbolises how deeply intertwined life and love are in nurturing our existence.

The third L, **Laughter**, must be paired with love to foster joy and happiness. Laughter without love can be harsh and damaging, potentially tearing relationships apart or leading to larger conflicts. But when laughter is infused with love, it creates warmth and joy.

The fourth L is **Labour**. Labour without love feels burdensome—like another day at work or endless chores. However, when your labour is driven by love, it feels blissful. It becomes the reason you're excited to wake up every day. I work with much more passion and less fatigue when doing my work and chores with love, not merely slogging through.

Lastly, the fifth L, **Listening**, becomes transformative when combined with love. Without love, listening is just hearing empty sounds, but listening with love? That's where true understanding and connection happen.

These Five L's—**Life, Love, Laughter, Labour, and Listening**—form my foundational philosophy. They guide how I approach my life, ensuring that each step is grounded in love and purpose, making the journey bearable, joyful, and deeply fulfilling.

I hope these principles can guide you, too, offering a sturdy framework for building your life, especially through transitions like menopause, where embracing a new phase with positivity and purpose can make all the difference.

My Tips for Transitioning into Menopause

If I could offer a tip to a woman entering menopause, it would be this: start seeking out the good things in life. Look for the light because you won't see it if you don't look for it. If you find yourself feeling stuck in a dark and harsh place, take a moment to pause and look around. See if there's a way to reach for something beyond the pain and suffering you're experiencing. Remember, you can choose how you respond to these challenges.

This isn't about theology; these are my thoughts. Think about when the earth was created—it was perfect. Humanity was granted dominion over this perfection, not domination, which is where we went wrong. Dominion means to care for. We mistakenly assumed we were meant to dominate, leading us to take more from Mother Earth than we should have. Now, we have a chance to reevaluate our relationship with the planet. If we love and care for it, the earth will reciprocate that love.

Find out more about Dr Gladys McGarey.

To connect with Dr. Gladys McGarey's wisdom and explore her work, visit the Foundation for Living Medicine at foundationforlivingmedicine.org. Founded to promote holistic health and well-being, her foundation advocates for a new healthcare paradigm that integrates mind, body, and spirit, empowering individuals to lead healthier and more connected lives.

Her latest book, *The Well-Lived Life: A 102-Year-Old Doctor's Six Secrets to Health and Happiness at Every Age*, along with her other publications, is available through major retailers.

Reflecting on our Conversation

The Importance of Honouring Our Elders

After my conversation with Dr. Gladys McGarey, it became clear that I was speaking with a living legend. Her presence was a reminder of life's vibrant possibilities, especially after menopause. Dr. Gladys is a true inspiration, showing us all how to live fully at any age. I see her as a keeper of time and wisdom, her hair neatly arranged like a crown earned through overcoming countless challenges and paving the way for future generations. Her willingness to share her story and inspire others to seek the light in their lives is a gift for which I am deeply grateful.

Writing her story reminded me how much we have lost by sidelining our elders. There was a time when elders were the matriarchs and patriarchs—the keepers of time, wisdom, and knowledge. They guided younger generations in healing their bodies, tapping into intuition, and navigating life's complexities. This wisdom, passed down through generations, was a living legacy shared within families and communities.

But today, we have drifted away from that path. Elders are often medicated, not always out of necessity, but because there's profit to be made. In the United States, nearly 90% of people aged 65 and older are on at least one prescription medication, and more than 66% take five or more. The pharmaceutical industry profits immensely, generating over $200 billion annually from drugs prescribed to this age group. Similarly, the aged care industry is booming, with the global eldercare market projected to reach $1.7 trillion by 2027. This industry is valued at over $300 billion in the U.S. alone.

This shift has led us to accept the misguided notion that ageing must mean decline and that losing our memories is inevitable. Yet those memories and the wisdom they carry are vital for guiding humanity. Elders have a crucial role but are often isolated in nursing homes, cut off from the communities they helped build.

In many cultures, elders are treated with the utmost respect and reverence. Countries like Japan, South Korea, China, and India have deep-rooted traditions that honour the elderly as wise custodians of cultural heritage. In Japan, for example, the elderly population is among the healthiest and most respected globally, with a strong cultural emphasis on honouring older generations. This respect and care keep them engaged and active in the community, contributing to Japan's high life expectancy of 84.63 years.

In contrast, in societies where the elderly are marginalised, life satisfaction and overall health tend to be lower. The loss of elder wisdom has left many feeling isolated and disconnected from the roots of their culture and history.

We need more voices like Dr. Gladys's, who share their wisdom and ensure we don't forget where we came from. We must remember the strength of the community and the guidance that only our elders can provide. The false sense of independence that encourages us to live in isolation weakens the very fabric of our society.

When one person in a family or tribe suffers, the collective once stepped in to help. But today, with our elders sidelined and our communities fractured, there is a lack of knowledge and wisdom. We must bring back the elders, honour their place in our communities, and learn from their experiences. If you have older people living near you, reach out to them. Offer them food and ask them to share stories about their past and how life used to be. We must keep those stories alive and continue learning from them.

Reconnecting with our elders preserves the past; it strengthens our present and future. It reminds us that true independence doesn't come from isolation but from being part of a community that values every member, from the youngest to the oldest. It's time to honour our elders, bring them back into the heart of our communities where they belong, and recognise their invaluable role in guiding us all.

If an elder in your life, like Dr. Gladys, wants to share their wisdom with the world, offer to be their camera and tech person. Dr. Gladys can share so much with us because of the support from her son, John, who helps bring her wisdom to a broader audience. A big thank you to John for sharing his mother with the world. Doing so can help rebuild the sense of belonging and wisdom that is so desperately needed in our world today.

Reflection Activities:
Embracing the Five L's

These activities help you deeply understand and apply Dr. Gladys McGarey's Five L's—Life, Love, Laughter, Labour, and Listening—into your daily life. These principles guide you toward connecting with your inner wisdom and enhancing your well-being. Through reflective questions and practical exercises, you'll learn how to weave these values into your routine, creating a more fulfilling and joyful existence.

Activity 1: Reflecting on Life and Love

Objective: Observe and appreciate the interdependence of life and love in the small moments of your day. Awareness of these moments will nurture a deeper connection between life and love in your everyday experiences.

Exercise: As you move through your day, consciously notice instances where vitality and kindness intersect— for example, holding the door open for someone or sharing a meaningful conversation with a loved one.

Reflections:

- How did focusing on life and love change your day's quality?

- Did you feel more connected to the people and world around you?

- Take a moment to reflect on how this awareness deepened your appreciation for life and love's interconnectedness.

Additional Action: Extend this principle to your community by checking in on an elder in your area. Listen to their stories with love and appreciate the wisdom they have to offer. This simple connection can be incredibly enriching for you and them.

Activity 2: Laughter with Love

Objective: Incorporate laughter into your daily routine to cultivate the joy and well-being it brings. Laughter, especially when shared with love, can reduce stress and foster connections with others.

Exercise: Find ways to bring more laughter into your life—watch a funny movie, attend a comedy show, or share jokes with friends. Ensure the humour is warm-hearted and inclusive, fostering positivity rather than harm.

Reflections:

- How did laughter affect your mood and interactions?

- Did it create a more joyful atmosphere and strengthen your connections with others?

- Reflect on how laughter, coupled with love, enhances your well-being.

Additional Action: Share a laugh with an elder by reminiscing about joyful memories or funny stories from their past. This shared laughter can bridge generations and bring immense joy.

Activity 3: Labour with Love

Objective: Transform mundane tasks by infusing them with love, making even the simplest chores feel meaningful and satisfying.

Exercise: Choose a routine task you find tedious. As you perform it, focus on how this labour serves you or others with love. Infuse the task with positive energy and intention.

Reflections:

- How did your perception of the task change when you approached it with love?

- Did you feel more connected and satisfied?

- Reflect on how a loving mindset can transform your attitude towards work.

Activity 4: Listening with Love

Objective: Develop mindful listening skills to enhance relationships and increase self-awareness by focusing on listening with love.

Exercise: Engage in three conversations where you focus entirely on listening. Don't plan your response; be present and absorb what the other person says.

Reflections:

- What did you learn from listening deeply?

- How did it affect your understanding and empathy?

- Reflect on how mindful listening can strengthen your connections with others.

Additional Action: Visit an elder and practice mindful listening. Allow them to share their life stories, wisdom, and experiences without interruption. Listening with love can create a powerful connection and honour the wisdom of our elders.

Activity 5: Personal Action Plan

Objective: Integrate the Five L's into your life on a regular basis to enhance your overall well-being and happiness.

Exercise: Create a chart or journal entry outlining how you'll incorporate each of the Five L's into your weekly routine. Be specific about your actions and how you'll remind yourself to live by these principles.

Reflections:

- How do you expect these practices to improve your well-being?

- Reflect on how committing to the Five Ls can shift your approach to life and health.

Additional Action: Incorporate a regular check-in with an elder into your plan. Make it a habit to visit them, listen to their stories, and learn from their wisdom. This can enrich your understanding of the Five L's and strengthen community ties.

Conclusion:

Reflect on the activities and insights gained from these exercises. Consider how integrating the Five L's might shift your approach to health and wellness. Keep a journal or notes to track your progress and notice any changes in how you feel physically, emotionally, and spiritually over time.

By embracing these activities, you're enhancing your life and reconnecting with the wisdom of our elders, who are the keepers of time and knowledge. Now more than ever, we need their guidance. So, let's open our hearts, share our stories, and speak with love. Let's honour our elders and bring their wisdom back into the fabric of our lives.

CHAPTER 2

Ibu Robin Lim

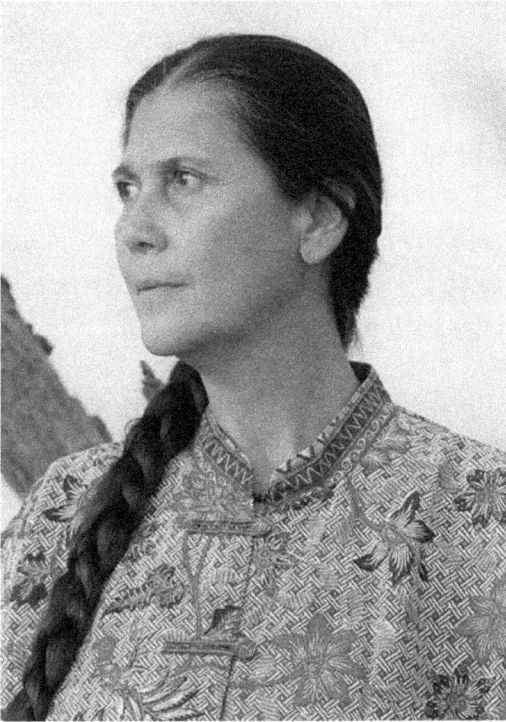

The Mother

Discovering Ibu Robin Lim

Discovering Ibu Robin Lim's book The Placenta: The Forgotten Chakra, I realised how little I knew about the placenta's importance, even after giving birth to two children. My knowledge of the placenta had been entirely medical, but Robin's book opened my eyes to its spiritual relevance throughout pregnancy.

In her book, Robin mentioned that the placenta is similar to a chakra, an energy centre in the body. This idea matched my experience with yoga and crystal sound healing, which involved the chakra system, and this increased my curiosity in her work.

I now understand the role of the placenta in our spiritual path from birth and our journey in life. Before, I had only thought of the clinical side of childbirth, but her point of view exposed a more spiritual part of it. This sparked my interest in understanding how the process of birth influences our entire lives.

Robin is a Filipino-American who lives in Indonesia. Her diverse background provides a unique perspective on women's health. Her experiences have broadened my understanding of menopause and deepened my appreciation for various cultural approaches, leading to a greater respect for human diversity.

Robin's work has opened my eyes to learning how our bodily and spiritual lives are connected. It has helped me understand the importance of how we enter the world, which enormously influences how we journey through life.

Background of Ibu Robin Lim

Lovingly known as 'Mother,' Ibu Robin Lim is an internationally known midwife, writer, and maternal health activist. She offers women and their families gentle, compassionate, and holistic care through the Bumi Sehat Foundation in Bali, Indonesia. By combining traditional birthing practices with modern medical knowledge, Robin has redefined the standards of maternal healthcare.

Heritage and Culture

Robin's diverse ethnic background, with a Filipino mother and an American father, influences her approach to midwifery and women's health. She values ancient knowledge and natural processes as essential to respecting the body. Her unique background allows her to integrate wisdom from multiple traditions, resulting in a practice that resonates with women from various backgrounds.

Worldwide Appreciation and Recognition

In 2011, CNN named Robin the 'Hero of the Year' for her tireless dedication to maternal health. This recognition of her influence on maternal and child welfare drew attention to the Bumi Sehat Foundation. Robin has established multiple community health and birthing facilities in Indonesia and the Philippines through this foundation. These facilities provide a safe space for natural birthing and comprehensive women's care.

Publications and Support for Maternal Health

Robin Lim is an accomplished writer. Her books, including *After the Baby's Birth*, *Placenta: The Forgotten Chakra*, and *Eat Pray Doula*, mix scientific study, cultural knowledge, and useful guidance to enable women to reclaim their birthing experiences. Every book shows her dedication to teaching healthcare professionals as well as women. Her next book, *The Yoni Owner's Manual*, is to offer insight into embracing the sacred feminine.

Daily Life and Relationship to Her Work

Robin is a mother and devoted grandmother. Her experiences have given her empathy and understanding, which enable her to help women at all phases of life. Robin supports women's respect for their bodies. Her approach highlights the value of community, ancestral knowledge, and learning to enjoy every phase of life. Working with her helps one to access sometimes neglected areas of female strength and well-being.

"Every baby's first breath on Earth could be one of peace and love.

Every mother should be healthy and strong. Every birth could be safe and loving. But our world is not there yet."

Ibu Robin Lim

A Conversation with Ibu Robin Lim

What is Delayed Cord Clamping and a Lotus Birth?

My children were born at home under the guidance of a midwife. We used delayed cord clamping and cutting the umbilical cord until after the placenta was delivered for all my children.

This helps increase the iron levels in the newborn by helping the placenta's blood to be sent to the baby, providing essential nutrients. Among other health benefits, this method reduces the risk of anaemia and enhances general health and development.

We also practiced Lotus Birthing, in which the baby's umbilical cord is not cut straight away. Instead, it naturally detaches from the baby three to ten days later.   This approach allows the baby to remain connected to the placenta, promoting a gentle separation. Lotus birthing is believed to have both symbolic and spiritual significance.

At Bumi Sehat, a health facility catering to families in Bali, Indonesia, we delay cord clamping and cutting for several hours until breastfeeding is well-established and the woman feels comfortable. This approach helps the baby make the most of the blood from the placenta, enabling their passage to life beyond the womb. It also enables the mother and baby to bond through skin-to-skin contact and breastfeeding, contributing to a positive postpartum experience.

Placenta Traditions in Bali and Indonesia

In Indonesia, there are specific traditions related to the placenta. Families bring the placenta home and give it a proper burial in observance of the child's guardian angel. Every child is believed to have a guardian angel, regardless of faith. This angel resides in the placenta during gestation and is thought to keep the mother and the baby alive by providing nutrients and oxygen.

The placenta is truly a miracle of nature. From a scientific perspective, it is astonishing how it filters and uses the mother's blood, even when it may be a different blood type. This incredible organ transfers essential nutrients and oxygen to the developing baby and removes waste products. The placenta's functions are essential for enabling the health and development of mammals during reproduction.

Natural Cord Detachment

Some parents choose not to cut the umbilical cord of their newborns and instead allow it to detach naturally. However, this practice is not for everyone and depends on family preferences. For example, in the case of my granddaughter Joanna, we allowed the placenta and umbilical cord to stay intact with baby, and then burned the cord to sever it after about 30 hours. I have noticed that giving the placenta a name may delay the natural separation. My grandsons, Bodhi and Tashi, both had 'Full Lotus Births,' meaning we did not cut the cord and allowed for the detachment to happen naturally after three days.

Once a baby is born, if the umbilical cord is not cut until after the placenta if born, so that one can see and experience the trinity of baby, umbilical cord and placenta, that is already what I consider a 'Lotus Birth.'

After the birth, if the family chooses 'Full Lotus Birth,' we clean the placenta with water, preserve it in coarse sea salt, wrap it in towels, and place it in a basket. This odourless approach provides a gentle transition for the baby, mother, partner, and other family members.

In this traditional practice, children in the family stay close to the newborn after childbirth, waiting for the cord to detach from the placenta naturally. When it finally falls away, the children joyfully run outside to play and share the news with the neighbourhood. The community honours this moment, recognising it as the soul's transition, intertwining with the newborn's earthly life. This guardian angel, believed to be present from birth, remains with the child throughout their life, providing support and protection.

Like you and me, every child is thought to have a guardian angel. This guiding presence watches over us, safeguarding our journey through life and gently assisting us when it's time to transition from this world.

Cultural Significance and Safety

The tradition of honouring the placenta has deep roots in Balinese and Asian cultures and holds significant importance in Filipino culture, which I learned because my mother is Filipino. The cover of my book *The Placenta: The Forgotten Chakra* showcases a photo of a baby named Wishaka still connected to his drying placenta in a basket, taken about two and a half days after his birth. Wishaka was born into my hands, and his uncle, Dr Pariatha, an obstetrician-gynaecologist (OB-GYN), supported the practice of full lotus births, which involved not cutting the umbilical cord at all.

Many people believe leaving the placenta attached after birth is unsafe. However, I know two (OB-GYNs) who left their children's cords intact until they naturally fell off three or four days later with no adverse effects. This practice is also common in Indigenous cultures. Ethnographic evidence suggests that many cultures have historically embraced this approach. Renowned primatologist Jane Goodall has even shared photographs showing apes walking around and breastfeeding their babies with the placenta tucked under their arms.

The Importance of Waiting

Allowing the umbilical cord to turn white before clamping and cutting it is crucial. This natural process may take around 15 minutes or up to three hours as the cord continues to pulse. Leaving the cord intact until it has finished pulsing provides oxygen and nutrients for the baby. During this time, the mother needs to have skin-to-skin contact with the baby, facilitating the baby's first embrace of life. Midwives, doulas, and (OB-GYNs) who advocate for natural birth highlight the significance of this practice, asserting it is a human right for the baby to have their first embrace and receive all the well-documented benefits that come with delayed cord clamping.

Changing Policy for Delayed Cord Cutting

In the past, I struggled with managing my anger, which affected my ability to advocate for babies and their placentas effectively. As I matured, I learned to approach situations with a calmer mindset. We needed to push for change to prevent trauma for newborn babies, who are the most vulnerable members of our society. Things became more manageable once I calmed down and let go of my anger. It all fell into place when women and their partners realised the truth.

Hospitals' policies on cord clamping and cutting are currently undergoing significant changes. The World Health Organisation now emphasises the benefits of delaying the clamping and cutting the cord as the preferred approach. This achievement follows 26 years of persistent efforts to advocate for change, leading to a single-word modification in the Indonesian midwifery manual. Previously, the manual mandated that the umbilical cord be clamped and cut immediately after birth. The transition from **'immediate' to 'delayed'** represents a significant milestone in this long-standing endeavour.

The recent changes in maternity care represent a broader shift toward a more natural and compassionate approach to childbirth. By emphasising the importance of the placenta and advocating for delayed cord cutting, we aim to encourage more hospitals to implement practices that provide every newborn with the best possible start in life.

My grandmother often shared stories with me of when she would attend births. She was a traditional midwife in the mountains of the Philippines before, during, and after World War II. She attended births in the mountain villages and would return the next day after birth. If the family wanted to remove the placenta, she would use her own cigar to burn off the umbilical cord. Sterile instruments were not available, but by not cutting the cord in those conditions, the baby remained unharmed and avoided the risk of infection. This approach was traditional but probably changed over time when women stopped being the primary caregivers of other women.

Reflections from Shivam Roshana

Australian author and birth keeper Shivam Roshana deeply moved me. While I wrote *Placenta: The Forgotten Chakra,* Shivam released her book, *Lotus Birth.* I received a copy from Jeannine Parvati Baker, a renowned author in conscious conception and prenatal yoga. Shivam Roshana's book completely captivated me, and I could not put it down.

Shivam Roshana wrote, 'In modern medicine, we throw the baby's placenta in the trash. Remember, the placenta is genetically identical to the baby. So, you had a twin, I had a twin—we all had a twin in our placenta growing in our womb. It was not just a piece of meat. It was our organogenesis, and it was pulsing. We played with the cord; we hugged it. It protected us, communicated with us, gave us everything we needed and took away everything we did not need. Then, suddenly, thrown in the trash. How many people in Western culture spend decades feeling like trash?'

Reflecting on Roshana's words, discarding the placenta represents a significant departure from how we respect the important connection between mother and child. This modern approach can leave people feeling disconnected and undervalued, echoing a deeper societal issue that deserves thoughtful consideration and change.

The Loss of Tradition

My mother often shared her experiences with me. She talked about how her mother worked as a traditional midwife and how different her experiences were in North American hospitals after marrying an American man. She felt that women received no respect during pregnancy, childbirth, and postpartum in those hospitals. Everything was very clinical and sometimes cruel.

When my mother had her children, she was far from everything familiar and dear to her. She was given injections to stop her from breastfeeding me and my siblings, which was very upsetting for her. The injections were meant to prevent breastfeeding and maintain a youthful appearance, preventing aging. This led to a loss of wisdom and history that elderly women could pass on, as they no longer played an important role in society.

However, this was not the case in every culture. In Indonesia and the Philippines, elders are not sent to care homes to be forgotten. Instead, they continue to be involved in their communities, respected and valued for their wisdom and contributions.

This history offers tangible evidence of why the role of elderly women was diminished. The fear created by witch hunts made it difficult for women to form supportive relationships, which still affects women today, making it hard to fully embrace the wisdom and knowledge that comes with age.

Embracing the Role of the Crone

As we age and gain wisdom, our responsibilities transition from caring for infants in our wombs and breastfeeding to extending care beyond our immediate families. We become crones—keepers of time—a role of immense significance.

Historically, elderly women, known as 'crones,' were marginalised in European culture, and this trend significantly influenced North America. During the witch-burning era, many women avoided reaching the crone phase altogether. To illustrate this, imagine a scenario: my pregnant neighbour on a farm gives birth. As an eldrly, postmenopausal woman, I prepare a meal for her family, help with laundry, clean her house, and care for her. However, somehow, men got the idea that these nurturing actions led people to label women like me as witches. The simple act of compassion and support was misconstrued as witchcraft.

Any display of care from an elderly woman toward a younger one could result in accusations of witchcraft. This fear shattered the trust between women. Caring women were burned as witches or drowned with stones tied to their bodies. Women were conditioned into believing that supporting other women could lead to death. This conditioning is ingrained in our genetic memory, and this historical trauma has impacted how women interact and support each other today. It took our generation to challenge this fear finally.

The role of the crone today involves reclaiming our place as the keepers of time and wisdom. It means nurturing not just our families but our communities as well. By supporting each other, sharing our wisdom, and providing care, we dignify the essence of being a crone. This transition is not just a personal journey but a collective one, restoring the bonds between women and reclaiming our rightful place as powerful members of society.

Intergenerational living

We share our home with my 92-year-old mother, surrounded by her great-grandchildren daily. Our family dinners are at 5 o'clock, which works perfectly for the little ones. This allows them to have baths, read books, and go to bed at a reasonable time. The schedule also suits my mother, who prefers to eat early. Organising our family life around our youngest and eldest members, particularly my mother, ensures everyone stays connected and supported.

Respecting and protecting the process of childbirth and the wellbeing of mothers and babies is crucial, as they are vulnerable. Equally important is to respect elderly women, often called 'crones,' for their significant roles in the community. In Indonesia, elderly women ensure the care of children, enabling their adult descendants to pursue education and contribute to the family's prosperity. Maintaining this rhythm keeps us intact and strengthens us as a family, enabling us to handle difficult times together.

I often feel disheartened when I hear some women say, 'I don't babysit,' when they become grandmothers. They are not just babysitting but embracing the role of an elder. Encouraging children to be around you helps build a strong sense of community.

My grandchildren can visit me anytime at Bumi Sehat, our clinic in Bali that provides free community health services, including childbirth, physiotherapy, acupuncture, lab analysis, ambulance transport, cryotherapy for early stages of cervical cancer, prenatal and elders yoga, breastfeeding support, youth services, and more. This interconnectedness spans four generations and provides a strong support system for children and elderly people.

Living in an extended family in Bali means that children have access to multiple grandmothers, which helps create a sense of safety and continuity. For example, when my mother's blood pressure rises, a simple hug from one of my grandchildren can help regulate it.

Embracing our roles as crones allows us to support our families and communities, pass down wisdom, and maintain connections across generations. This practice enriches our lives and strengthens the bonds that hold us together.

Graceful Aging and the
Challenges of Menopause

Growing up with my Filipino grandmother, I witnessed how gracefully she handled aging, and my mother followed in her footsteps. The only time my mother experienced significant difficulty during menopause was when my sister tragically passed away due to a childbirth complication caused by a doctor's negligence in Alabama.

The maternal mortality rate in the U.S. has been increasing since 1986 despite significant investment in childbirth technology. This statistic became personal for me when my sister, Christine, a woman of colour who was heavyset, passed away at 32. Her death was preventable, she had healthcare insurance and saw her OB/GYN asking for help with her symptoms of eclampsia, only hours before her death. The doctor brushed my sister's concerns aside, when he should have immediately hospitalised her, considering her symptoms indicated a life-threatening condition. Our Family was deeply impacted.

During this challenging time, someone suggested that my mother visit an OB-GYN, even though she had been managing her mild menopause symptoms on her own. She followed the advice and was prescribed medication. The stress from my sister's death, combined with the medication, caused her to transition from managing menopause well to experiencing severe bleeding, debilitating depression, and a significant disruption of her serotonin levels. The medication had varying negative effects on her well-being.

Witnessing her suffering, I convinced her to gently wean herself off the medication. Although she had only taken it for a few days, it took about a month to return to her graceful state. My own experience was much like my mother's, I focused on eating wisely and was fortunate to experience an even smoother menopause. Our family genetics have been kind to us in this regard—my mother remembered her grandmother Maria Flora in the Philippines also having a beautiful menopause.

Not every woman experiences a smooth menopause, and that's completely normal. No one should feel guilty if they find it challenging. I was fortunate to have the support of many women and men, including midwives, who offered guidance. While working at Bumi Sehat, I regularly received acupuncture, had time to rest, especially during heavy bleeding, and was well-nourished. My husband was incredibly supportive; he cooked most of our meals, so I didn't have to worry about that. Being surrounded by supportive family and colleagues at Bumi Sehat, our nonprofit foundation and clinics predominately staffed by women, helped me through this transition.

I also found that embracing my new role as a crone, a keeper of time, and recognising the fullness of my power provided spiritual and psychological support. Understanding and accepting this truly helped me navigate through my menopause with strength and positivity.

Sweet Potato Medicine for the Uterus

My grandmother always said, 'Whether you're in your childbearing years, trying to conceive, pregnant, postpartum, perimenopausal, or postmenopausal, eat sweet potatoes.' In Aotearoa, which is present-day New Zealand, Indigenous peoples held sweet potatoes as a sacred food.

In the last seven years of her life, at the age of ninety, my grandmother moved to America to be closer to my mother. Despite living in poverty in the Philippines, my grandmother selflessly gave all the food to the children— not only her great-grandchildren but also all the children she helped bring into the world as a traditional midwife.

When she arrived in the US, the first thing she did was plant a large, sweet potato garden. She believed they needed real fire to cook properly, so she would wash the sweet potatoes outside and cook them in the fireplace. This unconventional cooking method frustrated my American father, as he couldn't understand why a woman in her nineties would squat by the fireplace cooking meals in our house in California.

When my children were young, they spent a lot of time with their great-grandmother, who taught them everything about sweet potatoes. She showed them how to cook, grow, and harvest sweet potatoes and even how to use the leaves as leafy greens to increase their iron intake. According to her, sweet potato souls have reincarnated on Earth to nurture us, especially women and children. Sweet potatoes are medicinal for the uterus. I have found that when I eat them, I feel stronger, and my experience with menopause seems easier to manage. So, grow your sweet potatoes and enjoy them. They are inexpensive at the farmer's market and available in grocery stores worldwide.

Becoming the Crone

In my time as a midwife, grandmother and going through my menopause while supporting other women, I have come to realise that menopause is an 11-year process. It's not something to rush through in a set timeframe. You understand we are all on a spectrum when you see it this way.

As our children grow, and our responsibilities change, we have time to explore new interests. These might involve writing, painting, creating a peaceful home environment, gardening, sculpting, singing, composing music, wood carving, and making beautiful quilts. We can accomplish a lot more when we don't rush through menopause.

In this stage of life, we become crones—positive and vital members of society. Our responsibilities shift from focusing on our immediate family to engaging with the broader community. Whether we share wisdom through writing articles, express it through art, or create uplifting gardens for those passing by, these roles are incredibly important. This 11-year peri-menopausal span is when we truly embrace these changes.

We start as maidens, and when we do our maidenhood well, taking care of ourselves, allowing ourselves to be students and growing with the nurturing of our mothers and the wisdom of our grandmothers, we transition into motherhood. As we grow into motherhood, we hopefully have strong support systems that enable us to care for our children effectively—this includes support for breastfeeding. Women don't fail at breastfeeding—it is the support systems who fail mother and child.

Each stage builds upon the previous one, and skipping a stage is not an option. By embracing each phase—from maidenhood through motherhood to becoming a crone, we can be burnished into life's most golden phase, wise womanhood. By dancing through each of life's phases gracefully—we lay a sound foundation for the next generation.

The Keepers of Time

The constant news feeds on our devices inundate us, making it hard to escape. Society is facing challenges, and the world is in turmoil and in need of healing. As elders, who are the guardians of time and keepers of history, we are responsible for moving forward and shaping a positive future. Unless we respect our elders and grandparents as valued members of our society, rather than placing them in nursing homes, we cannot achieve balance and harmony. By recognising and appreciating the wisdom of our elders and by showing them love and care, we can contribute to lasting peace on Earth.

I recently had a wonderful conversation with my young female Balinese assistant. Her father is Trunyan, making her Bali Aga, one of the most Indigenous people in Bali. During our conversation, she shared her thoughts on patriarchy and amazed me with her wisdom, which she credited to her grandmother and great-grandmother. These traditional Indigenous Balinese women taught her that patriarchy is a failed experiment. They believe we must embrace the strength of our matriarchal lines to uplift men.

Capitalism is not functioning. While it may benefit a few wealthy individuals who aren't concerned about the future, it fails to serve everyone. We have lost the sacred rituals of celebrating ourselves as women, recognising our children as souls, and returning the placenta to Mother Earth when it falls away.

In Balinese culture, the most important life-worshipping ceremony is when a child touches Mother

Earth for the first time. This reflects the relationship between your earthly mother and Mother Earth.

If we can raise children by respecting their placenta, returning it to the Earth when it falls away, and recognising the child as a soul, respecting each stage of womanhood—from maiden to mother, to crone, to a wise woman—we will achieve lasting peace. We must protect our planet because there is no alternative, Earth is our one and only home. My granddaughter wears a T-shirt that reads, 'No music on a dead planet.' Every young person I speak to is deeply worried about the state of the planet and whether they will have a place to call home.

Appreciating the divine feminine in all stages is essential for creating a harmonious home. Respecting the crone is the missing piece of the societal puzzle today.

My Experience Through Menopause

Our bodies undergo a tremendous and beautiful change during menopause, and it's crucial to honour that. When my daughters began menstruating, which in Bali we call 'datang bulan' or 'the moon is here,' I taught them to view this time as their resting period. My daughter would say, 'I'm resting,' embedding this respect into our family language. This same respect extends to menopause—recognising the need for rest and creativity. We must learn to accept the ebb and flow of what our bodies tell us daily.

When I went through menopause, I experienced symptoms as well. Starting menopause around age 57, I remember missing periods and, by fifty-eight, had gone through twelve cycles without one menstruating. During this time, I experienced heavy bleeding on two occasions. Acupuncture helped manage these episodes of clots and bleeding, and I rested. In our family, when a woman releases blood—whether young, a mother, or elderly—she rests.

I had friends who suffered from severe hot flushes. While I experienced mild hot flushes, I embraced the heat as part of my journey. I was happy to be at this stage of life, supported by my village, the staff at Bumi Sehat, and my family.

In Bali, respecting the natural changes in a woman's body is deeply ingrained in our culture. We celebrate and observe these changes. Menopause is natural, beautiful, and embraced—not rushed through or dreaded.

Reflecting on these experiences, I believe women should celebrate each stage of their lives. Each phase—maidenhood, motherhood, and cronehood—builds upon the previous one, laying a firm foundation for the next. This is especially important in the Western world, where becoming a crone is not celebrated as it should be.

Learning from Our Ancestors

If you delve deeply into your family history, you will find wise women—keepers of wisdom—who have supported each other through childbirth and all stages of life. Our grandmothers were seekers of wisdom, and we all have that lineage somewhere in our ancestry. One practice I strongly encourage is tracing your female lineage.

My daughter, whose father is Chinese, traced her ancestry back seventeen generations with the help of her Chinese grandmother. I can only trace back five generations. Many women in the United States struggle to name their great-grandmothers or great-great-grandmothers due to lost knowledge of earlier generations. This discovery process has brought us closer, connecting us deeply with our roots and giving us a sense of belonging and continuity.

We have limited detailed records of my father's side, but my Filipino mother's side has a more well-documented history. Every day, I call upon them, saying, 'I'm calling on my placenta angel and my ancestors to come close to me, to guide and protect me.' This simple ritual of acknowledging their presence gives me strength and guidance.

If you go back far enough, all women will find wise women in their lineage—keepers of wisdom—helping others through birth and all stages of life. Our grandmothers sought wisdom, and we all have that strength somewhere in our background and ancestry. Researching your family history deepens your connection with your roots, brings a sense of continuity and support.

Many cultures worldwide have unique practices for honouring their ancestors, reflecting a universal human desire to stay connected to our roots. Whether through ceremonies, rituals, or simply remembering their names, these practices strengthen our sense of identity and community.

A Love Letter to Your Placenta

I want to share a personal practice I recommend to all women: reconnecting with our placental angels. Many of us feel disconnected unless we know where our placenta is buried or how it was memorialised. I felt the need to address this in my life.

When I was writing *Placenta, the Forgotten Chakra*, the spirit of my placental angel was distant. I wrote a letter to my placenta as a soul, apologising for the circumstances of our separation—how it was severed and discarded at my birth, leaving its spirit confused and traumatised. I also apologised for my inability as a baby to control what happened to us and for my mother's loss of power, being so far from her culture and her mother.

I invited my placental angel to come closer and stay with me because I needed its presence. I placed the letter with incense sticks and flowers in my garden and set it all alight. This act of sending my message through fire and smoke was my way of reaching out, mending that bond, and seeking forgiveness and closeness with my guardian spirit. It was a healing moment that I believe can offer similar healing to others who undertake this reflective and therapeutic action. Since our placenta nourishes us during our gestation, I observed that after writing the letter to my placenta, my relationship with sources of nourishment, for example, money, became so much better.

What Gives Me Joy?

My grandchildren bring me the greatest joy. I am also inspired by the remarkable women I work with from all over Indonesia and the Philippines. Also, the doulas and young midwives attending our Bumi Sehat seminars. At Bumi Sehat, we teach them to provide gentle, respectful care. We believe that skilled medical care is essential, but it must also be spiritually gentle, encompassing all aspects of life—from birth and motherhood to perimenopause and even the portal of death.

My relationship with my husband has evolved beautifully as I have stepped into my role as a crone and wise woman. I was fortunate to marry a man who respected and loved his mother deeply, and I always tell my daughters, 'When choosing a partner, find someone who respects and loves his mother.' This is foundational not only for your relationship but also for honouring your menopause.

Five Tips for Navigating Menopause

Eat Lots of Sweet Potatoes: Sweet potatoes are a fantastic food for this stage of life. They are nutritious and have been a staple in many cultures for their health benefits. Our family considers sweet potatoes as medicine for the uterus. Including them in your diet can provide the nutrients your body needs during this transition. For instance, my husband often roasts sweet potatoes, which we enjoy with some butter, making for a comforting and nourishing meal.

Connect with the Earth: Walk barefoot on the grass. Take off your shoes and feel the connection with Mother Earth. She is our mother and home and is crucial in helping us through this process. Earthing helps circulate energy and keep us grounded. This practice can bring a sense of calm and balance during a significant change. I remember feeling overwhelmed; walking barefoot in the garden gave me peace and reconnection.

Seek Out Your Female Friends and Ask for Help: In Western society, seeking assistance is challenging due to our isolated lifestyle. I have observed cultural differences, having lived in the Philippines, Bali, Hawaii, and America. I have built a support system of female friends who understand and can offer help when needed. We all support our daughters to rest during their menstruation.

Embrace Traditional Practices: Medicine has deep roots in traditions that support women in all life stages, including menopause. When I was in Bali during the postpartum period, everyone cooked for me and served me. I was told not to go to the kitchen while I was bleeding after giving birth, as it was my resting time. This experience was wonderful, and we should embrace and honour the tradition of caring for new mothers.

Embrace Your Zest: Margaret Mead said it best: **'There's nothing more powerful than a postmenopausal woman with zest.'** Embrace this phase with zest and wisdom, knowing you are entering a powerful and transformative time.

Find Out More About Ibu Robin Lim

To learn more about Ibu Robin Lim, her compassionate work in maternal and child health, and her training programs, visit the Bumi Sehat Foundation at bumisehat.org. Founded by Ibu Robin, Bumi Sehat provides gentle, respectful maternity care, particularly for underserved communities, and advocates for the wellbeing of mothers and babies worldwide.

If you're interested in training as a doula, Ibu Robin offers the IPE (International Postpartum Education) Doula Program, which includes advanced training for those wanting to expand their knowledge and skills in holistic maternal care.

Her latest books, *Bali, A Cage in Paradise* and *The Yoni Owner's Manual*, are available for purchase on her website, iburobin.com, along with more information on her work, writings, and resources for doulas, midwives, and caregivers.

Reflection on my Conversation with Ibu Robin Lim

Community vs Independence

After speaking with Robin, I realised how much her story resonates with me. Growing up in a close-knit Indian community in London, I witnessed first-hand the power of communal living and mutual support. I remember how mothers would support one another when a child was born. The younger generation cared for the grandparents while the grandparents cared for the young, and there was no concept of paying for a babysitter. The entire community would come together in times of crisis. But now, I find myself questioning the path we've taken—the push toward independence and self-sufficiency that has, in many ways, left us more isolated.

We live in our little boxes, often not even knowing our neighbours. This isolation, this so-called independence, can feel particularly heavy for a new mother. Without the community's support, motherhood can be an incredibly lonely journey. That loneliness is compounded by the absence of the multi-generational wisdom, joy, and playfulness that should accompany childhood.

I felt this loneliness as a first-time mother living on the other side of the world from my family. It was a solitary experience, and I longed for the support that used to come so naturally within a community. When I reached my perimenopause years, it was the first time I consciously sought out the support of other women. I turned to the wisdom and knowledge of the women featured in this book, reaching out online to find the guidance I needed to navigate this significant transition in my life.

In many ways, this journey has brought me full circle— I am seeking the connection and communal support that once surrounded me, even if it's in a different form.

The Role of the Crone

In modern society, especially within Western culture, we have become disconnected from the wisdom of elder women, known as crones. These elder women have experienced maidenhood and motherhood and now find themselves on the threshold of their crone years. Unfortunately, these women are often disregarded as nothing more than irritable old ladies, but this perception is far from the truth.

The crone embodies wisdom accumulated over a lifetime, a wisdom that comes from seeing with the heart and soul. Her intuition, honed by years of experience, is sharp and deeply attuned. Yet, instead of honouring these wise women, we often place them in care homes, isolating them from the community they could be nurturing, as Robin pointed out.

Sadly, our society has forgotten how to respect and learn from our elders. We've lost sight of the value they bring and the knowledge they hold. Perhaps it's time to bring the crones back into the leadership roles in our communities, to help humanity remember how we're meant to live and to guide us back to a life connected with the wisdom of the ages.

Menopause: A Continuation of Our Birth Journey

This conversation has left me reflecting on the increasing rates of intervention in childbirth, and something feels unsettling. It appears something essential is missing—whether it's love, care, or a deep understanding of the beauty that comes with motherhood. Yes, motherhood can be challenging, but it's also filled with incredible, life-affirming moments. The fear that some women now feel about giving birth seems unnatural, especially considering that childbirth is the most natural act, one that women have been doing for thousands of years without intervention.

How we enter this world has lasting effects on the rest of our lives. Robin's work highlights the importance of returning to and remembering how childbirth used to be—a process supported by wise women who carried the knowledge and experience of generations. These women assisted in births with a deep, innate understanding of the process.

Just as we navigate childbirth, we also navigate our transition into menopause—a process that marks the birth of our new role as the crone, the wise woman. We should turn to the crones to learn how to embrace this role, stepping into it with our heads held high, ready to share the wisdom we've gathered.

The Market for Placentas

Curious about the placenta's significance, I delved into research and discovered that it is highly valued in both the medical and cosmetic industries due to its rich content of stem cells, growth factors, and hormones. These components are used in regenerative medicine and high-end skincare products.

There is significant demand for human placentas in China and the United States, particularly in Traditional Chinese Medicine (TCM) and the cosmetic industry. In TCM, placentas are believed to boost the immune system and improve reproductive health, driving up demand and prices. In China, fresh placentas are sold for around USD $70, while processed pills cost about USD $157 per bottle. Interestingly, placenta from male babies is often priced higher due to a belief in their superior strength and vitality. In the United States, high-end skincare products containing placenta extracts can cost hundreds of dollars. Placentas from C-sections are especially valued for their perceived cleanliness, as the placenta has not gone through the birth canal, increasing their demand and price.

I have been left wondering about what happened to the placenta of my children after my hospital births. I cannot recall being asked permission to use it for medical research. Additionally, I wasn't informed about how it was disposed of. Society's obsession with youth raised questions about whether it was sold for purposes like cosmetics. Furthermore, I wondered if the high demand for placentas might contribute to the increasing rate of caesarean sections in hospitals.

Letter to My Placenta

Following Robin's advice, I wrote a letter to my placenta. A deeply personal and transformative experience. As I put pen to paper, I realised I was connecting with a part of myself that had been long neglected. This acknowledgment was healing, reminding me to embrace every aspect of ourselves.

Robin's wisdom has inspired me to navigate each stage of life with grace and gratitude. It has deepened my understanding of the natural transitions of a woman's body and the spiritual significance of childbirth. Her insights have also expanded my perspective on the vital role of community and the wisdom passed down through generations.

Now, more than ever, I am committed to cultivating a sense of community, supporting women through every phase of life, and honouring the wisdom of our ancestors. By seeking guidance from our guardian angels and quieting our minds, we can reconnect with our inner wisdom and trust in the support that surrounds us.

Embracing My Purpose

Like Robin, I realised I have also been 'hijacked' by a higher purpose. The universe has guided me to write this book, to explore these truths, and to share them with you. When it is time for knowledge to emerge, the universe chooses you, takes you on a journey, and temporarily hijacks your life.

Reflection Activity: Embracing Menopause, Honouring Our Ancestors, and Finding Joy

Inspired by Robin Ibu Lim's insights, this activity sheet is designed to help you navigate menopause, reconnect with your spiritual roots, and honour your female lineage. These activities offer practical advice, emotional support, and spiritual enrichment, strengthening your connection with your body, ancestors, and the natural world.

Activity 1: Incorporate Sweet Potatoes into Your Diet

Regularly add sweet potatoes to your meals—roast them, make soup, or include them in salads.

Reflect:

- Write about how different foods make you feel and note any changes in your well-being after incorporating sweet potatoes.

Activity 2: Connect with the Earth

Spend at least 15 minutes daily walking barefoot in your garden or a nearby park. Focus on the sensation beneath your feet and your connection to the Earth.

Reflect:

- Write about your feelings of calm and balance after each session and how this practice helps you feel more grounded.

Activity 3: Gather with Female Friends

Arrange regular meetings with your female friends or join a women's circle. Share experiences, support each other, and enjoy nourishing foods together.

Reflect: Consider how these connections enhance your well-being and document your reflections.

Activity 4. Create Personal Rituals

Establish a monthly rest day or create a special ritual to mark significant life transitions. This could include taking a relaxing bath, meditating, or setting aside a day for rest.

Reflect:

- Note how these practices support your journey and bring you peace.

Activity 5. Write a Letter to Your Placenta

Find a quiet space, reflect on your relationship with your placenta, and write a letter to it.

Reflect:

- Apologies for any past neglect, invite its spirit to guide and protect you, and perform a ritual to symbolise reconnection and healing.

Activity 6: Research Your Family History

Gather family records and talk to elderly relatives to trace your female lineage.

Reflect:

- Document your journey and discoveries and consider how learning about your ancestors impacts your sense of identity.

Activity 7: Acknowledge Your Ancestors Daily

Incorporate a daily ritual of acknowledging your ancestors, such as lighting a candle or saying a prayer.

Reflect:

- Write about how this practice provides strength and guidance and how it enriches your life.

Activity 8: Find Joy in Life

Spend quality time with loved ones and engage in activities that bring you passion and fulfilment.

Reflect:

- Journal about these experiences and how they contribute to your happiness and well-being.

CHAPTER 3

Alexandra Pope

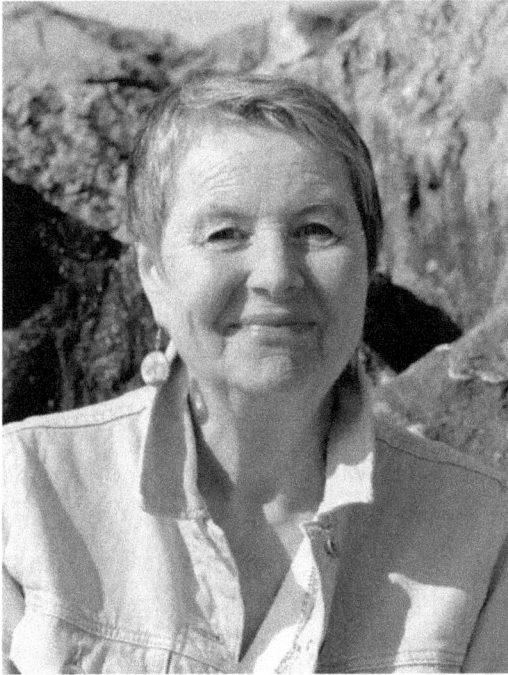

The Initiator

Discovering Alexandra Pope

When I first encountered Alexandra Pope's work, it felt like a light illuminating a path I had long been searching for. At a time when I was yearning for a deeper connection to my body, her teachings on menstrual cycle awareness and the transformative power of menopause provided exactly what I needed. She gave voice to thoughts and feelings I had struggled to articulate for years.

Even before discovering Alexandra, I had instinctively attuned to my body's natural rhythms, observing changes in energy, mood, and creativity throughout my cycle. Unbeknownst to me, I was already practising what would later be called menstrual cycle awareness—the practice of paying attention to the physical, emotional, and spiritual shifts that occur throughout the menstrual cycle and using that knowledge to align your life with those natural rhythms. This practice grounds us in our bodies and offers a way of understanding ourselves as individuals and as women.

This intuitive connection began in my early twenties when I briefly used the pill for contraception. Despite being on it for only a year or two, something inside me knew it wasn't for me. The artificial control over my cycle felt out of sync with my body's natural flow, and stopping the pill was the first step toward trusting my body's wisdom, even if I didn't fully understand it at the time.

As I deepened my understanding of menstrual cycle awareness, I realised how we are initiated into womanhood—through our first bleed, or menarche—shapes the rest of our journey into womanhood. Whether we are taught to embrace or ignore our cycles can influence our relationship with our bodies and ourselves. If this initiation is one of shame or suppression, we often carry those feelings into adulthood. But when we are encouraged to honour and respect our cycles, we develop a healthier, more empowered connection to our womanhood. Understanding this helped me see my own journey in a new light and gave me the tools to reframe my past experiences.

As I learned more about menstrual cycle awareness, I began to consciously work with my body's rhythms, using them to enhance my life. For example, during my time in the corporate world, I scheduled important meetings during ovulation, when I felt most confident. As my menstruation neared, I carved out time for solitude, reflection, and recharging. I adjusted my physical activities, swapping intense workouts for gentler practices like yin yoga during menstruation. These intentional shifts had a great effect on my well-being. It wasn't until I immersed myself in Alexandra's teachings that I realised I had been tapping into ancient wisdom all along.

Her work validated my experiences and empowered me to live in harmony with my cycle rather than against it. Alexandra reframed the menstrual cycle as a biological process and a source of spiritual insight. Her teachings deepened my understanding of the practices I had already been using and helped me see them as tools for reclaiming the power that society often diminishes in women. This new perspective enhanced my professional life and strengthened my respect for my body's natural rhythms.

The more I explored her teachings, the more I understood how important her work is—not just for me but for women everywhere. Alexandra and her co-founder, Sjanie Hugo Wurlitzer, have a unique ability to connect with the deepest aspects of womanhood, bringing them to light in a nurturing and empowering way. Their emphasis on the cyclical nature of life, especially through the transition of menopause, resonated deeply with me. It was a timeless and revolutionary perspective, reminding me of the power we harness when we align with our body's natural cycles.

When I began writing this book, I knew I wanted to share the wisdom of extraordinary women who have dedicated their lives to uplifting others. I am grateful that Alexandra agreed to be part of this project. Her willingness to share her journey, insights, and guidance with you, the readers, is a true gift.

I hope that, through her words, you will discover the strength and power that comes from embracing the natural rhythms of your body and life. Have you noticed how your energy shifts throughout the month? Perhaps you're already in tune with your cycle without even realising it. Let Alexandra's teachings help you engage with this wisdom more consciously and see how it can transform your life.

Introduction to Alexandra Pope

Alexandra Pope is a pioneer in the emerging field of Menstruality and the co-founder of Red School, an organisation dedicated to empowering women by helping them reconnect with the natural rhythms of their menstrual cycles. With decades of experience and a background in psychotherapy, Alexandra has become an expert in using the menstrual cycle as a tool for personal growth, creativity, spirituality and leadership.

Through her own experiences with her menstrual cycle, Alexandra recognised its transformative potential. This discovery led her to develop (along with her colleague Sjanie Hugo Wurlitzer) the concept of menstrual cycle awareness, which has since become the foundation of Red School's comprehensive educational programs and resources. Her work emphasises the cyclical nature of women's lives and bodies, advocating for societal change in how women are supported—from their first period to menopause.

Along with her co-founder, Sjanie Hugo Wurlitzer, Alexandra has co-authored influential books such as *Wild Power: Discover the Magic of Your Menstrual Cycle* and *Awaken the Feminine Path to Power and Wise Power: Discovering the Liberating Power of Menopause to awaken Authority, Purpose and Belonging.* These works guide women to embrace their menstrual cycles as a source of strength and spiritual insight. She has also co-authored *The Pill: Are You Sure It's for You?* with Jane Bennett, exploring the physical, emotional, and mental effects of hormonal contraception while encouraging informed choices that align with the body's natural rhythms.

Central to Alexandra's teachings is the belief that understanding and honouring the menstrual cycle can lead to spiritual awakening, deeper purpose, and a sense of personal authority. Her work has inspired countless women to embrace their natural rhythms, leading to more empowered and fulfilling lives. Through fostering community and offering support, Alexandra has become a guiding light for women navigating the often complex and beautiful journey through menopause.

As you explore Alexandra's journey and insights, you will uncover the transformative power of menstrual cycle awareness and the changes that come with embracing the wisdom of menopause. Her story is not just one of personal growth but a call to all women to reconnect with their innate strength and wisdom during this transitional phase of life.

"Menstrual cycle awareness is the missing key to understanding

our health, creativity, and spiritual life as women."

Alexandra Pope

A Conversation with Alexandra Pope

My First Bleed

I was meant for this work from the moment I was born. Something was always guiding me, but it truly began with an awakening during my first period—my menarche. From that moment, I somehow knew that the menstrual cycle was something wholesome to be honoured. I never felt any shame around it, and I realise now how powerful that was.

Like many young women in my early 20s, I went on the pill. But I didn't stay on it long—something inside me strongly resisted, and I knew it wasn't right for me. Thankfully, I listened to that instinct. However, I still needed contraception, so I began exploring fertility awareness. By 24, I was charting my cycle and knew exactly when I was ovulating. This practice connected me deeply with my body and was incredibly empowering.

Surprisingly, I had been tapping into something profound without even realising it. At 29, I wrote in my diary, **'The world is singing today. Last night, I got my period.'** That's the spiritual force of menstruation at work. I felt alive and vibrant. My entire being seemed to wake up with the bleeding, but in my innocence, I hadn't yet made the connection. I hadn't realised that menstruation is an altered state of consciousness. I had been honouring my cycle in a somewhat unconscious way.

The Big Awakening
Managing Pain

The big awakening moment came just before my 31st birthday. I was living in Sydney, Australia—had only been there for a few months—when I started experiencing the most excruciating menstrual pain. It was utterly shattering, lasting three to four days each month. That's when I decided to listen to my body truly. I thought, **'My body is talking to me, and I will listen.'** Surgery and drugs weren't my path, so I turned to natural therapies, which I was already interested in. This decision marked the beginning of a deeper, more conscious connection with my body and my menstrual cycle.

I gave myself space to rest during menstruation. This wasn't easy—I had work and responsibilities—but I did my best to make it happen. It didn't always work out perfectly, but I made space whenever I could, and as a result, I rarely needed to take medication. Instead, I chose to face the pain head-on, going cold turkey. There was something about that experience that lifted the veil from my eyes. During menstruation, I rested to reduce stress on my body and mind. This was an important part of my healing process. I learned to pay attention to my cycle, track when menstruation was due and organise my life around it. This was an early version of what we now know as menstrual cycle awareness.

How it all began?

I felt like my menstrual cycle was leading me, determined to heal me at all costs. My initial workshops took place at Sydney's Royal Hospital for Women, which was still in Paddington before it relocated to Randwick. I approached the health education centre there, and an enlightened nurse who managed it said, 'Why not?' Despite being a psychotherapist and not a health educator, I felt compelled to initiate these workshops. I identified those who would be interested in learning about menstruation – specifically those who were struggling with it. This is precisely how it all began: women struggling with menstrual issues attended, and I taught them how to honour the rhythm of their cycles.

Piece by piece, everything started to make sense. We started with a basic map of the different phases of the menstrual cycle, and from there, we discovered other maps and teachings that helped us understand the power of the cycle even more. This whole journey came from my own deeply felt experience of healing. I paid close attention to myself, and the cycle revealed its wisdom to me through that. We aren't taught to connect with our cycles, but a whole inner world opens when we do. It felt like my menstrual cycle was trying to get my attention by sending me pain that forced me to stop and listen. And in that silence, I could uncover new perspectives and see another world.

Managing the Pain of Discomfort

How did I manage the pain? I went cold turkey—moving my body, feeling the pain, and leaning into it. I often used my voice, stretching, and doing yoga—deeply engaging with my body to ease the pain. My partner at the time was extraordinary; he would hold me and rock me through the pain while I cursed the patriarchy. He met me where I was and held me as I faced the pain fully.

As I changed my diet, I became so familiar with my body and the pain that I could immediately tell if something I ate affected me. For example, one time, I thought, 'Oh screw it, I'm going to have a life,' and went out for a decadent breakfast with friends at a harbour café. That day, I ended up in the emergency room at King's Cross Hospital, getting a heavy-duty painkiller injection. I knew then that I had pushed myself over the edge but learned from it. Each month brought new lessons; through those lessons, I grew more connected to my body and its wisdom.

The Calling That Changed Everything

I was following my passion, fuelled by an unconscious force that seemed to be leading me. It's hard to pinpoint the exact timeline, but I remember feeling an undeniable 'call' from menopause at forty-eight. Even though I didn't experience menopause until I was about fifty-three, it felt like menopause was already sending me a message:

'You're going to change everything in your life, and this is what you're going to do.'

I had the realisation that I should quit being a therapist and return to the UK. Initially, I thought, 'Wow, how is that even possible?' I had lived in Australia for 18 years; by the time I left, it had been 25 years. I was self-employed and had established a life in Australia. However, I decided to take a risk. I thought, 'All right, I'll go to England to visit my family and start holding workshops while I'm there.' And that's exactly what I did. During each visit, I would arrange a workshop or two, and everything started to unfold.

The Serendipitous Meeting with Sjanie

I first met Sjanie during one of my early workshops in the UK. It might have been the first workshop I ever had there. At the time, we didn't particularly connect. Then, out of the blue, Sjanie contacted me later with a question about psychotherapy. She knew what I had studied and was trying to decide her path.

I remember this happening when I planned to return to the UK. Casually, I told her, 'By the way, I'm going to be moving back to the UK.' To my surprise, she quickly replied, 'Oh, we must get together.' It was total serendipity that she reached out to me at that moment.

When I returned to the UK, I reached out to as many people as I could since there wasn't an established foundation for my work there. I had to start from scratch, except for a few workshops I had done and a small group of people who had experienced them. Sjanie and I connected during a meeting, and our conversations flowed smoothly. Our initial meeting led to more discussions, and we began brainstorming ideas together. She casually suggested, 'Why don't we collaborate on a workshop?' I thought, 'Sure, why not? Let's do it.' From there, one thing led to another, and that's how it all started.

Red School slowly began to take shape naturally from our collaboration. We have been working together for approximately 16 years now. After going through various iterations, Red School was officially incorporated seven years ago. We had a different name before Red School, but each step led us to where we are now.

Menstrual Cycle Awareness Preparation for Menopause

Menopause wasn't an issue for me because I was already immersed in the wisdom of cyclical consciousness. Each month during menstruation, I experienced a mini death and rebirth—a microcosm of the larger transition I would later go through at menopause. These monthly experiences were like training wheels, preparing me for the big journey ahead.

Menstrual cycle awareness helped me grow into myself, deepening my inner knowing, authority, and power. It awakened the meaning of my life—my calling. I was steadily evolving into who I was meant to be, which continued throughout my life. Menopause became the final chapter in this journey that began at menarche. It brought everything to fulfilment, allowing me to fully become the person I was meant to be and to serve my true purpose. My post-menopause years are the harvest of all the fruits of my cycle awareness, cultivated over time as I evolved into menopause.

In my 40s, I never used the term 'perimenopause.' Instead, we use the term 'The Quickening' because I didn't want people to think of themselves as being in menopause when they're really in a transition. When people say 'perimenopause,' they often mistake it for menopause itself, but it's a period of preparation. I didn't give menopause much thought because I was so engaged in living my life and exploring the existential questions that came with it. I knew that the fulfilment of who I was would come after menopause.

Self-Caring While Expanding My Work

During this time, I worked as a psychotherapist. Although I excelled in this role and had a strong practice, I had a nagging feeling that it wasn't my true calling. I wasn't necessarily unhappy, but I sensed that there was something more meaningful for me to pursue. My menstrual cycle constantly reminded me that I was meant for something greater. Each month during my period, I felt the power of this cycle, which fuelled my desire to expand my work.

While continuing my work as a psychotherapist, I also began leading menstrual workshops, giving talks at psychotherapy conferences about the menstrual cycle, and teaching about it to students and natural health practitioners. I was deeply immersed in my life while also prioritising self-care due to severe health issues, including menstrual problems and chronic fatigue. Being ambitious, I was often frustrated by the lack of energy that held me back. Therefore, I made it a priority to maintain my health and keep moving forward.

Navigating Exhaustion and the Call of Menopause

In my 30s, I experienced night sweats, but that was due to adrenal fatigue. At the time, I could have easily labelled it as early menopause and panicked, thinking, 'Oh my God, I'm already going into menopause, and I'm just 39!' But thankfully, that wasn't my mindset back then; menopause wasn't even on my radar the way it is for many today. I was exhausted—completely worn out from adrenal exhaustion—so I focused on addressing that.

When my menstrual cycle became irregular in my early 50s, I initially didn't attribute it to menopause. Instead, I was preoccupied with deeper questions about my life. At the age of 48, I suddenly felt a strong directive from within—almost like a message from menopause itself—telling me to give up my therapy practice and return to the UK. Despite my initial doubts about how to make this happen with limited resources, I eventually decided to listen to that inner voice and make the necessary changes.

I love the idea that the universe takes you over, sorts you out, and gives you instructions on what you need to do for the sake of the world. You have to surrender to it because it's out of your hands. That's the wisest advice you can give anyone going through menopause: surrender completely.

So, I received my instructions, and I set my intention. I didn't tell anyone—not even my mother—because I didn't want to set any expectations. And the rest is history. It took me seven years, but eventually, as I was coming out of perimenopause, my feet touched the soil of the UK. That marked the beginning of something new—a whole new chapter in my life.

Interestingly, I didn't have hot flushes at all during menopause. I remember wondering, 'Is that a hot flush? I'm not sure.' I didn't experience them. The only time I started having sweats again was after I got to the UK, and that was due to the exhaustion of moving countries. So, once again, it was adrenal exhaustion.

The Seasons of the Menstrual Cycle and Life

Menstrual cycle awareness is like the seasons of the year. It's all deeply interconnected. We often talk about the different seasons within the menstrual cycle. Menstruation is your inner winter, pre-ovulation is your inner spring, ovulation is the summer of your cycle, and pre-menstruum is the autumn of your cycle.

But there's more to it than just the monthly cycle. We also consider the seasons of your entire menstruating life. From menarche (your first period) through your 20s, you're in the spring of your menstruating years. From your late 20s and through your 30s you're in the summer of your menstruating years. All the qualities we associate with these seasons—renewal, growth, energy—are echoed in the monthly cycle and the broader journey from menarche to menopause.

Then, in your 40s, you enter the autumn of your menstruating years. This is why many people feel the pre-menstrual energy more during this time—a tougher energy, more critical and sometimes reactive side can become more dominant. But it's important not to abandon the other qualities of your menstrual cycle during this phase. Finally, as you reach the end of your 40s, you enter the winter of your menstruating years, menopause.

Menopause: Entering The Inner Winter

Menopause is like wintertime; you're going deeply inside yourself. I love this analogy because if we think about winter in nature, it's when nature sheds its leaves at the end of autumn. Similarly, as you approach menopause, you start shedding things.

I remember culling my library to a third of its former glory, giving away things I no longer needed. You may find yourself stepping back from certain friendships or responsibilities. It's extraordinary—you're preparing to step away from the world.

During winter, nature rests and undergoes deep reparation beneath the surface while everything appears quiet on the surface. This rest and rejuvenation allow for new life to bloom in spring. In modern agriculture, we often neglect this natural need for rest, constantly pushing the soil to produce by adding more and more chemicals. But true sustainability requires honouring that need for rest and renewal, allowing things to regenerate. The same is true for our bodies and souls during menopause. We're entering our inner winter.

The Challenge of Letting Go

As you approach menopause, you start letting go of the things that once seemed so important, the things that once floated your boat. If you have children, you might think, 'I love you, but can you just leave home now? Never mind that you're only ten years old! I've got other business to attend to, thank you very much.' Even with your partner, it can be challenging if they don't understand what's happening. It's not that you don't have love or understanding—you do. But this is the nature of menopause at work, and sometimes, our partners can feel like they're being rejected. The reality is, it's not about them. It's about you needing to step away and take care of yourself. But if people don't understand this process, they naturally feel hurt or rejected, and that's entirely normal. I would feel the same way if no one explained it to me.

This is why partners need to do their work, too. No one is a victim of menopause itself — we're all victims of a lack of understanding about it. If we truly knew what was happening, if we understood that this is a time of spiritual awakening, we would see that we need to step away from the world a bit, to let go of some of the pressures and responsibilities we carry, so that this spiritual awakening can take place with more ease.

The Awakening and Trauma

Experiencing a spiritual awakening is a big deal. We're talking about deep, transformative spiritual forces at work here. You must be prepared to receive it, to feel it, and to understand it. This kind of work demands something significant from you. It's no wonder there's so much trauma around menopause—many people don't realise that this spiritual work is calling them. They try to continue life as usual, showing up at work, performing the same roles, and being there for their family while another force demands their attention. These two worlds clash, and the result is often trauma—complete shutdown or exhaustion—because our energies are waning, and our culture doesn't value or appreciate older people.

The fact is, we all get older—everyone, across all genders. No one escapes aging. But we live in an ageist society where people desperately try to hold on to their youth. When you're also dealing with the aging process, it's easy to feel overwhelmed. You might think, 'Hang on a minute, I'm not going to follow that path,' because people are so caught up in staying young.

Many people don't realise that spiritual work is a calling. Instead, they try to keep living as before, working, caring for their families, and maintaining the same pace. However, this clash between the old way of life and the new spiritual demands can lead to exhaustion and even shutdown.

The Challenge of Aging and the Need for Rest

Dealing with getting older can feel overwhelming, especially in a society where everyone seems determined to cling to their youth. The trauma around menopause often stems from our failure to acknowledge and value the power and wisdom that older people bring to the table. This is a very real and toxic issue in our world.

As you experience menopause, your body is completely rewiring itself physically, which demands a lot of energy. There will be times when your brain and body need to adjust, and it's no wonder you might feel like shutting down. And honestly, that's exactly what you need to do. You want to close the curtains, shut the front door, turn off the world, and lie still in the dark. That would be ideal, but we live in a society without space for this kind of rest. We're not supported in taking that time for ourselves.

The challenge of menopause is finding the space to rest and reset. However, that won't stop me from changing the conversation around this. I feel passionately about this because we can't keep going the way we've been. I'm talking about the whole planet here—because we're exhausting nature by not valuing cyclical consciousness. Everyone is getting burnt out because we're constantly in 'on' mode, with no breaks and no time to rest. This angers me. It's no surprise we're facing a mental health crisis— this relentless pace leads to exhaustion and burnout.

The concept of cyclical consciousness is fascinating because it emphasises the importance of both activity and rest. It's similar to the wisdom of the circadian rhythm, which we all begin to recognise. Just as we need to sleep at night without compromise—no other medicine can replace the benefits of a good night's rest. Sleep is medicine, and nothing else can take its place. This rhythm holds a deep wisdom and is fundamental for our well-being. The same principle applies to the menstrual cycle and the different phases of our menstruating years. Menopause is a time for rest.

1% of Change – The Small Moves

What does rest look like when you still have to work, earn an income, or care for young children? It comes down to the power of small moves, small shifts. We talk about the 1% change. Your ideal scenario might be to stop working, step away from everything, leave your phone at home, and escape to a South Sea island where no one can reach you. You want to lie on the beach, have no one to care for, and just be. That's the dream. But realistically, we're aiming for 1%, maybe just half an hour in your day or week where you take time solely for yourself and are absolutely, categorically unavailable to anyone else.

Once you start doing this, something shifts in your psyche. A sense of dignity begins to return, self-affirmation starts to awaken, and suddenly, you begin to have radical thoughts. In that space, you're finally able to listen to yourself. You can't hear what's happening inside as long as you're constantly doing. **Listening to yourself is the true medicine for menopause.** You're being guided through this spiritual initiation, but to hear that guidance, you have to create the space to listen.

The Power of Saying No
Facing Your Truth

During menopause, you may start having thoughts and feelings that could create difficulties in your relationships. You might think, 'I'm not sure I want to continue this marriage,' or 'I need some time for myself.' Even though you care about your partner and don't want to hurt them, you may also think, 'I'm tired of taking on most of the parenting responsibilities. I need my partner to step up and do more. I'm overwhelmed with everything I must handle at home and want to do less. I want to change how things are done around here.'

These thoughts are inevitable, and you'll need tough conversations with your family. My book has a great story about an Italian woman, a classic Italian mother, who had started working part-time. This allowed her some sacred time to think while driving, and she realised that things had to change. So, she called a meeting with her husband and two teenage daughters and said, 'Things are going to be different. I won't be there for you like I used to be.' The teenagers were squirming and pleading with their dad, 'Can't you put something in her tea?' (Their dad happened to be a doctor.) They were desperate because she was withdrawing some of her services, and everyone else had to step up.

During menopause, there's a line you'll cross where you just can't push yourself anymore. A power arises—the power of saying no. You'll find yourself saying no to things before your brain can censor them. 'No, no, no, I can't do that. No, no.' It might sound negative, but it's not. You don't know what you do want yet; you only see what you don't want. And that's the beginning.

No one likes causing trouble, I certainly don't. However, there comes a point when your well-being will suffer unless you dare to speak up and ask for what you need. It's about opening up your heart and throat chakras.

Building the NO Muscle

When you start saying no, it might come as a shock to you and those around you. But as you keep saying no, it empowers you. Each no gets stronger and more intentional. With each no, you build up your 'no muscle', that's you asserting your boundaries. Menopause pushes you over the line, and suddenly, no pops out of your mouth, and you think, 'Whoa, where did that come from?' And then you realise, 'Oh, I rather like that.'

This is the biggest part of the early stage of menopause. You start facing everything you haven't fulfilled in your life up to this point—all the griefs you hold, any historical wounds or abuses in your system. It's all coming up for reckoning and healing.

This is not the time to judge or criticise yourself. It's a time to feel, embrace, and acknowledge all this. Let go of things that didn't or won't happen now. Something new is trying to emerge within that release—your true calling. You're letting go of what's not you and doing much deeper inner work.

The Inner Work and the Freedom to Be Myself

You confront some hard truths about yourself when engaging in deep inner work. I vividly recall coming face-to-face with my arrogance. I remember thinking, 'Wow, I was so arrogant.' Realising how much of a know-it-all I had been was quite confronting. I didn't want to lose my confidence, but there was a sense of arrogance surrounding it that I needed to acknowledge. And that wasn't all. Much anger surfaced as I began to see all the ways I had censored myself—all the ways I had denied who I truly was. I faced how I had tried to be something I wasn't, abandoning parts of myself in the process. But I confronted all of that and accepted it as part of who I am.

This inner work is vital. It's the medicine you need to prepare the true channel of yourself, the strong, coherent, authoritative channel that allows spiritual forces to flow through you and guide you. This is where the universe— or the 'hijack,' as Ibu Robin Lim, who is also featured in this book, beautifully put it—steps in. The hijacking drops you into a space where you're forced to do this inner work, aligning yourself with who you truly are. And when that alignment happens, it's a spiritual blessing.

You feel it in your very being. It's like, 'Oh, this is who I am.' It can be a quiet, gentle realisation or hit you suddenly. I remember one time I was walking down the street, and it just hit me—I slapped my forehead and thought, 'Oh my God, this is who I am.' It's funny to think about now, but it was such a powerful moment.

The Moment of Utter Freedom

When you reach that stage, it feels like pure, utter freedom to be yourself. I permitted myself to be my uncensored self. It was like, 'Oh God, yeah, what was I thinking? This is who I am. Oh, whoa, we're going for it now, unashamedly.'

Much of what holds us back is a shame, but when you truly solidify who you are, that shame starts to melt away. In that moment, your calling, your spirit, and the guidance from the universe can flow through you effortlessly.

I've always felt connected to my calling. I believe it began with my very first period—your calling does awaken at that moment. I had an extraordinary spiritual awakening while I was in boarding school, and there was something deep inside me working and guiding me even then. But now, after doing this inner work, that calling could fully take up residence within me. It could fill me, and I could finally get down to business and start manifesting it fully in the world.

The Vital Role of Community in the Menopause Journey

When it comes to navigating menopause and the role of community, I have two thoughts. First, community is absolutely essential, especially during what I call the 'death moment.' This is a time when you may feel deeply betrayed by life, which is why we refer to this first phase as Betrayal. You experience betrayal on many levels, and I explore this deeply in our book, *Wise Power*.

In that moment of betrayal, you may feel abandoned. It's a real life/death moment, and it's heartbreaking to see a rise in suicide rates among women at this stage. This increase is directly linked to feeling extremely abandoned and not understanding what is happening. At this time, it is important to have a supportive community that recognises this as a spiritual awakening—a community that respects your experience and truly understands you.

However, there is another side to this. While community is crucial, you do need help to do this work. It is essential to be seen, and if you need therapy or coaching, I highly recommend it. But ultimately, no one else can save you from this feeling of abandonment. This is the moment where you have to decide whether you're going to say yes to yourself—to who you truly are—or whether you're going to give in to all the opposing forces telling you what you should or shouldn't be, in effect abandoning yourself.

This is the spiritual initiation moment. It is important to have a supportive community that fully understands this. It is crucial to have post-menopausal women in this community because only they can truly grasp that no one else can save you. Others may try to intervene and improve things for you, but they should not. They cannot make it better. They can offer support as therapists and coaches do, but you need the presence of a post-menopausal woman who holds you in her gaze and says, 'I see you. You can do this. I can't do it for you, but I am the sentinel guarding you during this spiritual initiation.'

This thought makes me emotional because this kind of support isn't happening nearly enough. It would be the greatest gift to have older women and people who have gone through this journey who can hold this role with understanding. They've lived it and gone through it.

The World Needs Post-Menopausal Women

I believe the world desperately needs post-menopause women who have embraced their calling, who have been willing and sufficiently supported to face the darkness for a while—just long enough to do what they need to do. The awakening we undergo through menopause is also in service to the world. Who we truly are is what is needed for the world. Abandoning ourselves is like abandoning the world as well.

It's important to acknowledge that many people may think, 'After menopause, I just want a quiet life.' To those people, I say, 'Absolutely—go for it!' Living a quiet peaceful life, happy with who you are, is the gift you give the world. Just be happy, but don't become cynical. Don't let bitterness and cynicism take over because that would mean betraying yourself. Be kind, be happy, and stay true to yourself. That's the greatest contribution you can make.

The Force of Menopause

Since the dawn of time, menopause has been a spiritual awakening. What is changing now is our awareness and acceptance of it. It's almost like menopause is standing up and saying, 'I'm not going to stay quiet anymore.'

The potential impact of conscious menopause on serving the world is greatly needed. The menopause process seems to be evolving to meet the demands of our times. There is an unstoppable force at play here.

I would define that force as the Feminine—the archetypal feminine energy, the force present in all genders. I'm talking about the sacred feminine, the Divine Feminine, with a capital 'F.' This force has been forsaken for so long, but she is returning. It's unstoppable.

Menopause is such a potent, powerful channel for this resurgence. It's *the* channel, I would say, but this energy also speaks through other channels—nature, the menstrual cycle, and menstruation each month. People are being tapped on the shoulder by this energy in all sorts of ways, but menopause is the quintessential channel for the true, deep power of the Divine Feminine to flow through and be channelled back into the world.

The Joy of Creative Expression and Calling

I am filled with joy, even though managing an organisation is incredibly demanding. However, the work we are doing brings me immense joy. I see myself as an artist, and my art feels like my true calling. This work, focusing on menstruality, is not just a job; it's a calling. It's about serving the Divine Feminine and the ineffable through this work.

It's like being a painter with the genuine skill to create. My skill is the capacity to connect with the ineffable. These skills are precisely what's needed for this work and for everything we do at Red School. It's truly amazing to be completely in tune with who I am and to channel my gifts into the world.

It feels like an artist who has an idea for a creation and then brings it to life—painting the picture. I often find it amusing to read about famous artists. I'm thinking of David Hockney, the photographer who turned to painting. He's in his 80s now and keeps producing paintings. When you feel that death is close, you become so alive with what's important to you that you want to keep creating.

What brings me joy is having this channel to express my creativity in the world. For me, creativity and calling are interchangeable words. It's simply beautiful.

Tips for Embarking on the Menopause Journey

Tip One - Practice Menstrual Cycle Awareness.

If you're still in your 40s, my first tip is to practice menstrual cycle awareness today. Don't hesitate—do it. It's simple and opens up a whole new world for you. You can find out more about it on our website at RedSchool.net. Trust me, this is something you need to begin right now.

Tip Two - Listen to Yourself - Pay Close Attention

As you approach menopause, you might start feeling like you're going mad—but you're not—you're coming to your senses. Listen to yourself and pay close attention to your inner promptings. Hear, acknowledge, and take your inner thoughts seriously, but don't rush to act immediately. Instead, write them down and note those wild, radical, and random thoughts that drop in. You might not know what to do with them yet, but don't dismiss them because they're important.

Tip Three - Find Ways to Slow Down

In your 40s you'll enter what we like to call the 'quickening'. How you meet and tend to yourself during this time is everything in terms of your preparation for menopause. Then, as you move into the hinterland of menopause, things start heating up, and you realise, 'Okay, menopause is getting very "real" now. I can't deny it.' During this time, find ways to slow down your life. Start removing things that no longer serve you. Cull what you can.

Tip Four – Find Your 1% Time

The most important tip I can give you is this: you need time and space. This is crucial, and it's non-negotiable. I'm so fierce about this because it's not optional. You must find time and space for yourself, even if it's just 1% more than you're doing now. That small increase will make a big difference.

Tip Five – Get Serious about Self-Care

And finally, tend to your health. Self-care is everything because what you do today sets the foundation for your health post-menopause. Get serious about it—focus on good health practices, don't compromise your diet, and ensure you're getting enough exercise. What you do now will have a lasting impact on your well-being as you age.

Embracing the Journey Ahead

I want to emphasise that the journey through menopause is one of the most transformational experiences you will experience. It's a time to reconnect with yourself, to honour your body, and to embrace the changes with courage and grace. Remember, this is a journey that's uniquely yours, but it's also one that countless women have walked before you and will walk after you. By listening to your inner wisdom, making space for yourself, and tending to your health, you're not just surviving this transition—you're stepping into a new chapter of empowerment and self-awareness. So, take a deep breath, trust the process, and know you have the strength and resilience to navigate this incredible journey.

Where to Find Out More About Alexandra Pope and Red School

To learn more about Alexandra Pope and her work at Red School, visit redschool.net. Co-founded by Alexandra and Sjanie Hugo Wurlitzer, Red School is dedicated to menstrual cycle awareness and its ability to transform women's lives.

Red School offers a wealth of resources, including articles, workshops, and training programs, designed to support you in embracing menstrual cycle awareness as a powerful tool for personal growth, creativity, and spiritual awakening. Alexandra's books, along with additional resources, are available on the website, providing further guidance on your journey towards wellbeing, empowerment, and self-discovery.

My Reflection after Our Conversation

The Transition and the Pill: A Deeper Reflection

After my conversation with Alexandra Pope, I was struck by how deeply interconnected menstrual cycle awareness is with a woman's journey into perimenopause and menopause—what Alexandra aptly calls 'The Quickening.' This transition is not just a biological shift; it's a calling for women to step into their true purpose and embrace the life they were born to live.

As I reflected on this, I began to consider the impact of the contraceptive pill, which has become such a prevalent part of many women's lives today. Its influence goes beyond individual health, affecting relationships, lifestyle choices, and broader societal structures. Though I was only on the pill for a short period—less than two years—it led me to question its wider implications. Why has the pill become such a deeply embedded part of our culture, and what long-term effects might it have on women, particularly when used from such a young age?

The Economic Impact of the Pill

While studying financial planning, I realised how dramatically the introduction of the pill in the 1960s reshaped the global economy. Before the pill, most families in the West relied on a single income, with the husband typically working while the wife stayed home to care for the family. This arrangement made homeownership more accessible, as house prices were manageable on one income. However, as the pill gave more women control over family planning, many entered the workforce, and dual-income households became the new norm. This shift increased household income and consumer spending but also brought unintended consequences. As more families began relying on two incomes, house prices rose, making it difficult to afford a home on a single salary.

This shift toward dual-income households also altered family dynamics and societal structures. With both parents working, raising children increasingly fell to external childcare providers and schools, leading to the rapid growth of the childcare industry. In the UK, the childcare market was valued at £5.7 billion per year by 2020, and globally, the industry is projected to reach over $520 billion annually by 2030. As parents balance careers and family life, this growing dependence on external childcare reflects how the widespread use of the pill has enabled more women to enter the workforce, driving the demand for childcare services.

Furthermore, this shift created a feedback loop. As dual-income families became the norm, higher disposable incomes increased demand for housing, which drove up real estate prices. This made it nearly impossible for families to rely on a single income. As economic pressures continue to grow, we may see a resurgence of traditional family and community support systems, where extended families collaborate to sustain households. This could solve modern families' increasing challenges, giving parents more flexibility to balance work, childcare, and personal well-being.

The Financial Motive Behind the Pill

The financial aspect of the pill is significant. The global contraceptive market is enormous, with the demand for contraceptive pills alone projected to reach nearly $26 billion by 2026. The birth control industry is valued at approximately $37.5 billion, with the largest markets being the United States, China, India, Germany, and Brazil. Pharmaceutical companies have a vested interest in promoting the pill as a long-term solution, often encouraging women to start using it at a young age— sometimes for reasons unrelated to contraception, such as acne treatment—and to stay on it for decades.

A woman who begins taking the pill at 15 and continues until she's 55 has been a consistent consumer for 40 years. This longevity of use raises important questions about whether the promotion of the pill is truly in women's best interest or if it is largely driven by profit.

How the Pill Affects
Relationships and Partner Choice

Beyond its financial impact, the pill also affects women's personal lives, particularly their choice of partners. Research shows that hormonal contraception can alter a woman's attraction to certain types of partners. Typically, a woman's preferences shift throughout her menstrual cycle, with a heightened attraction to genetically compatible partners around ovulation. However, when a woman is on the pill, these natural hormonal fluctuations are suppressed, potentially influencing her partner's preferences.

One study found that women on the pill were more likely to choose partners with similar immune system genes. In contrast, those not on the pill were drawn to partners with dissimilar genes, promoting greater genetic diversity in offspring. This raises significant questions about how hormonal contraception may affect long-term relationships. For example, if a woman selects a partner while on the pill and later stops using it, her natural hormonal cycle returns, and her attraction to that partner may shift. Additionally, suppressing natural hormonal rhythms can dull a woman's intuition, making it harder to discern what she truly needs in a partner.

The Loss of Wisdom and Intuition

The pill's suppression of the menstrual cycle also means that women miss out on the natural wisdom and intuition that arise from being in tune with their bodies. The menstrual cycle is more than a biological process—it provides insight to guide a woman's decisions, emotions, and relationships. The deep connection to the self is often diminished when this cycle is artificially suppressed.

Many women who use the pill report mood swings, depression, and a sense of disconnection from themselves. This is because the pill interferes with the body's natural hormone production, which is crucial not only for physical health but also for emotional and mental well-being. By blocking the menstrual cycle, the pill can suppress the very intuition that women like Alexandra Pope encourage us to embrace.

I am grateful to Alexandra for helping me articulate this sacred knowledge. Her insights have given me the language to better understand menstrual cycle awareness, and I now feel more equipped to guide my daughters on their journey into womanhood, helping them stay connected to their bodies' innate wisdom. Our conversation brought me great clarity, for which I am deeply thankful.

This reflection isn't meant to dismiss the pill—every woman should have access to safe and reliable birth control. However, it's important to consider the broader implications of using hormonal contraception and to make informed decisions based on personal needs and circumstances.

A Call to Reflect and Research

Reflecting on these questions, I urge other women to do the same. If you are on the pill or considering it, take the time to research and understand what it truly does to your body, mind, and spirit. Consider how it might affect your mood, sense of self, and connection to your natural rhythms. Most importantly, listen to your intuition—the very thing the pill may be suppressing.

Let's start an open conversation about these issues, not to scare or shame anyone, but to empower women with the knowledge they need to make informed choices about their bodies. Menstrual cycle awareness is a powerful tool, and it's time to reclaim it as a source of strength, not something to be controlled or suppressed.

We are seekers of knowledge and wisdom. Do your research, question what you're told, and make the best decisions for yourself. I am simply sharing what I've learned on my journey.

Reflection Activity:
Your Menopause Journey

This activity sheet is designed to help you actively engage with the concepts discussed in the chapter and support your transition through menopause. By working through these activities, you'll gain deeper insights into your body, mind, and spirit as you navigate this transformative period.

Activity 1: Start Practising Menstrual Cycle Awareness

Why It's Important: Understanding your menstrual cycle helps you connect with your body's natural rhythms, which is crucial as you approach menopause.

How to Begin: Track your cycle daily, noting any physical, emotional, or mental changes. This will help you identify patterns and better understand your body's needs.

Activity 2: Listen to Your Inner Voice

Why It's Important: Your inner voice holds the wisdom you need during this transition. Listening to it will guide you through the challenges of menopause.

How to Begin: Reflect on your thoughts and feelings each day. Write them down, even if they seem random.

Over time, patterns will emerge that can guide your decisions.

Activity 3: Create Space for Yourself

Why It's Important: Menopause is when you need to prioritise yourself. Creating space allows you to recharge and listen to your inner needs.

How to Begin: Start by finding 30 minutes in your week when you are completely unavailable to others. Use this time for self-care, whether walking, meditation, or sitting silently.

Activity 4: Embrace the Quickening

Why It's Important: The 'quickening' phase in your 40s prepares you for menopause. Embracing this time helps you let go of what no longer serves you and make space for new growth.

How to Begin: Identify one area of your life to declutter—physical clutter, mental habits, or emotional baggage. Reflect on how this impacts your well-being.

Activity 5: Prioritise Your Health

Why It's Important: The habits you form now will support your health in the post-menopause years. Self-care is essential for long-term well-being.

How to Begin: Assess your current self-care routine and set small, achievable goals for improvement. Focus on areas like diet, exercise, and sleep, and make gradual changes to benefit your health.

Activity 6: Connect with Community

Why It's Important: A support network can make the menopausal transition smoother and less isolating. Sharing your experiences with others provides encouragement and perspective.

How to Begin: Reach out to others who are going through similar experiences. Join a local or online support group or start conversing with friends or family about your journey.

Reflection and Progress

At the end of each week, take some time to reflect on your experiences with the activities. Use your journal to answer the reflection questions and consider how these practices influence your understanding of menopause and overall well-being.

Remember, this journey is yours to shape. The activities are tools to help you connect with yourself and navigate this transformative time with greater awareness and empowerment. Be patient with yourself, and celebrate your progress, no matter how small it may seem.

Jane Hardwicke Collings

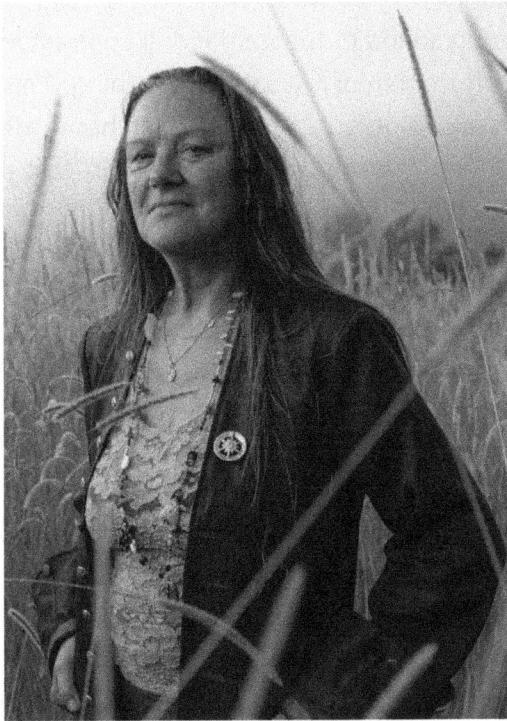

The Boss Witch

Discovering Jane Hardwicke Collings

As a first-time mother far away from my family's support, I recall the challenges and isolation I faced. One memory stands out: the day of a dentist appointment. I remember sitting in the dentist's chair, holding my six-week-old baby on my chest, the sharp, jarring sound of the dental drill contrasting sharply with the soft rhythm of my baby's breathing. This contrast intensified my vulnerability. As I walked home afterwards, tears clouded my vision, and the isolation cast a shadow over my journey into motherhood.

I longed for someone who understood this transformative experience, especially without family support. In my search for guidance, I discovered the work of Jane Hardwicke Collings, a midwife, teacher, and founder of the School of Shamanic Womancraft.

Jane is dedicated to empowering and aiding women in navigating life's transitions and shaping new beginnings from endings. Her teachings resonated deeply, offering a perspective that felt both ancient and affirming.

Jane introduced me to various techniques for embracing change, including delving into ancestral belief systems and shamanic rituals. For instance, she taught me how to perform simple rituals to honour the cycles of nature and my own life. Her teachings changed my perspective on motherhood and reshaped how I intended to approach menopause and prepare my daughters for adolescence and womanhood. I began to realise that my challenges were part of a broader issue experienced by women from generation to generation.

Reflecting on my own experiences, I recalled the shame of my first menstrual cycle. I fretted about potential stains on my bedsheets in the morning or menstrual blood leaking through my clothes during family gatherings or at school. I felt isolated and disempowered. Determined to ensure my daughter's experiences differed, I committed to teaching them that menstruation, childbirth, motherhood, and menopause are natural and beautiful aspects of life, free from shame.

As I transitioned from motherhood into menopause, I realised that both phases are significant rites of passage. Jane's teachings equipped me for menopause, another momentous change in a woman's life.

My journey from feeling isolated as a new mother to discovering a supportive online community highlights the importance of connection and shared wisdom. I found comfort and strength through Jane's guidance and the collective knowledge of like-minded women. This newfound community helped me realise that while I may have begun my motherhood journey feeling alone, embracing this support network has been crucial in shaping my approach to womanhood.

Introduction to Jane Hardwicke Collings

Jane Hardwicke Collings, founder of the School of Shamanic Womancraft, is an inspirational leader dedicated to empowering women through transformative practices. The school provides a supportive environment for learning and personal growth. Jane offers workshops, mentorship, and training programs rooted in shamanic practices. These programs honour women's experiences and promote a nurturing connection to the Earth and its natural cycles. Her teachings blend mystical, practical, ancient, and contemporary elements to create a comprehensive personal growth and empowerment approach.

She is the author of several books, including *Ten Moons: The Inner Journey of Pregnancy, Blood Rites: The Spiritual Practices of Menstruation, Becoming a Woman: A Guide for Girls Approaching Menstruation,* and *Herstory, a Womanifesto.* Jane's work is an invaluable resource for those navigating the sacred journey of womanhood. Offering guidance through physical transitions in life, they serve as a spiritual compass, helping women embrace their natural rhythms and reach their full potential.

Jane's philosophies emphasise life's cyclical nature and feminine empowerment. They invite us to dialogue with our inner wisdom and the larger forces at play in the natural world. Her teachings remind us of the power of honouring our natural rhythms and reclaiming the deep feminine wisdom that resides within us all.

As you delve into the pages ahead, I invite you to let Jane's insights inspire you to explore the depths of your being, embrace your cycles, and realise the fullness of your potential.

"Rites of passage are transformative events that guide individuals into

new phases of life, shaping their identities and roles within their communities."

Jane Hardwicke Collings

A Conversation with

Jane Hardwicke Collings
How It All Began

My Awakening to
Patriarchal Culture in Midwifery

I became a registered nurse at 19, completed my training at 21, and became a midwife at 25. During my midwifery training in a big city hospital in Australia, I had an unexpected awakening at 25. I wasn't expecting it because I didn't even know it was a thing. What I awakened to was the patriarchal culture. I hadn't realised what the patriarchal culture was as a 25-year-old back in 1984.

During my midwifery training, I witnessed institutionalised acts of abuse and violence being done to mothers and babies, masquerading as safety measures. I essentially woke up to the misogyny built into the maternity care services and the effects it was having on mothers and babies. This realisation deeply affected me and shaped my approach to midwifery and women's health, motivating me to seek and advocate for more compassionate and respectful birthing practices.

I completed my training and immediately left the hospital system. I could not stand by and be part of the damage. Seeing how mothers and babies were treated, spoken to, and coerced into non-evidence-based practices was too much. Sadly, things have not improved; in fact, they have worsened. Today, one in three women experiences birth trauma, and of these, one in ten develops Post Traumatic Stress Disorder (PTSD) as a result of their birth experiences. Alarmingly, 70% of these traumas are iatrogenic, which means that midwives and doctors—the very people who should be helping—are the ones who cause the trauma. However, there is a silver lining: we can change things. These service providers must do a better job and become conscious of their impact on women.

At 26, I made a drastic shift: I became a home birth midwife and dedicated the next 30 years to this practice. Home birth is a world apart from the mainstream; it is where families, especially women, take control of their bodies and their birthing experiences. Embracing this new role, I delved deeper into earth-based spirituality and shamanic practices, learning from many excellent teachers.

I continue the lineage of Jeannine Parvati Baker, a renowned teacher of women's mysteries from America. She passed away in 2005, but not before I promised—on her deathbed—that I would continue her work. This led to the founding of the School of Shamanic Midwifery. However, we had to change the school's name due to government pressure, which imposed substantial fines each time we used the original name.

I adapted and pivoted by renaming the school 'The School of Shamanic Womancraft,' a term from Jeannine that turned out to be a hidden blessing. This change expanded the school's reach, drawing in women of all backgrounds eager to start their transformative journeys. I have always embraced the term 'midwife' in its most original, traditional sense—to facilitate transformation and guide women through all stages of life, from womb to tomb.

My Journey into Menopause

I felt ready for my menopause, having already immersed myself in the spiritual practices of childbirth and menstruation. Viewing it through my midwife's eyes and heart, I saw menopause as another form of labour and birth. This perspective involved understanding the birth process and its impacts and highlighted how we can apply similar insights to menopause—as another rite of passage.

My extensive study and understanding of the rites of passage taught me that each transition naturally leads to the next. So, by the time I approached menopause, I fully grasped what rites of passage meant. I knew this phase would be a critical time to address and heal all the unresolved parts of myself. Dr. Christiane Northrup, M.D., a visionary pioneer and a leading authority in women's health and wellness, sums it up nicely, stating that whatever has been swept under the carpet will come out during menopause, a rite of passage designed to heal all unhealed parts. Armed with this knowledge, I entered menopause, ready to confront whatever came my way. Yet, the unhealed parts I encountered were challenging and confronting. Having done extensive research, I was well-prepared to recognise the recurring suppressive tactics against feminine power that are common in childbirth and menstruation and are now reappearing in menopause.

This transformational journey and its spiritual aspect presented a unique opportunity for healing—not just for me but also for the 'red thread,' the female generational trauma passed down through our mother line. This trauma also influences what we pass on to the younger women and men in our families, as the men learn from the women's experiences. I witnessed this unfolding in my menopause journey.

My Menopause Experience

I hesitate to use the word 'symptoms' to describe menopause because it is not a disease, despite often being mischaracterised as such due to hormone deficiencies or imbalances. Menopause should not be seen as a disease, so I prefer to call it an experience. This distinction is crucial for properly understanding and navigating this significant life transition.

Based on my own experience and that of many other women, one common issue during menopause is insomnia. It is best not to battle insomnia during this time. Instead of lying in bed and getting increasingly agitated because of the inability to sleep, it is better to use that time effectively. Many women, including myself, choose to get up at two or three in the morning to journal, write, or take part in other creative activities. This helps with healing through journaling and directs those nighttime energies towards productive pursuits such as writing books.

I have made some discoveries regarding my hot flushes. Similar to how someone might notice an aura before a migraine or an epileptic fit, there is also an aura to a hot flush. It is not commonly discussed, but adrenaline is released just before a hot flush. This surge of adrenaline sets the stage for the hot flush, and its impact heavily depends on your current level of stress and the general state of your nervous system.

Women, including myself, may experience a sudden feeling of impending doom and concern for their own well-being or that of their children as a result of the adrenaline release that accompanies a hot flush. This sensation, which lasts less than a minute before the hot flush begins, can be misinterpreted as anxiety. I found this particularly fascinating. During a hot flush, I might experience a toxic thought about myself or something else, which seems to be 'burned away' by the hot flush. This compelling analogy highlights the body's unique way of processing experiences.

The body communicates deeply, whether during the menstrual cycle, childbirth, or menopause. Our bodies are not simplistic; they are evolutionary miracles. Questioning what happens during menopause is like questioning the natural process of childbirth. These are all working systems, though they can sometimes cause discomfort or pain. However, the real issue often lies in the suffering that arises from the narratives we tell ourselves about these pains. Societal perceptions that paint menopause in a negative light have a significant influence on this story.

The Veil of Oestrogen

I have noticed that negative attitudes start early, even from our first period, leading to what is known as 'menstrual shame.' We are taught to see these natural processes as something to fear.

Around the age of 13, most girls experience their first period, known as menarche. This marks a significant shift in their hormones, leading to changes in their bodies and how they interact with the world. One of the most significant changes is the release of oestrogen, also known as the 'hormone of accommodation and self-sacrifice.' This hormone plays a crucial role in teenagers' lives, making them conform to their peers, dress like them, and blend in, often sacrificing their originality and personality to fit in with others.

As we enter our childbearing years or focus on growing our careers, projects, or businesses, the impact of oestrogen becomes more prominent. It compels us to prioritise the needs of others over our own. We often use phrases like 'Whatever you want, darling' or 'Let's do what's best for the children.' Even when hungry, we might say, 'I haven't eaten yet, but please go ahead.' If we run a business, we may put our personal needs aside, saying, 'I have to open the shop. People are relying on me.' Despite the personal costs, we are rewarded for this behaviour.

When discussing the 'healthy model' of navigating life phases, it is important to recognise that not everyone begins from the same starting point. Those who have experienced a traumatic childhood or adolescence often have to mature prematurely, taking on caregiving roles early in life, which significantly influences their life path; however, if we set aside these challenges and consider a scenario of a person transitioning into the mother or creatrix phase without such burdens.

In this healthier model, nurturing children, careers, or businesses can be incredibly fulfilling. There is an intense sense of reward when you see your children eating at the table, enjoying the nutritious meals you've thoughtfully prepared, or witnessing the success of a project or business you have poured your energy into. This fulfilment is a direct result of the self-sacrifice and accommodation dictated by the 'veil of oestrogen' that surrounds us during these years.

Around five years before menopause, which can occur at an unpredictable time, oestrogen levels begin to decline, and there is a shift in hormonal levels. First, progesterone levels decrease, followed by oestrogen. This hormonal shift can lead to significant changes in thoughts and behaviours. For example, phrases like '**How come I'm the only one who does anything around here?**' may start to surface, indicating a shift from a hormone-driven inclination to accommodate others.

Many women experience the changes as making them more aware of their needs, desires, and contributions, perhaps for the first time in their adult lives. This self-awareness can bring about significant changes, especially in relationships, as women question their roles and seek greater reciprocity and fulfilment.

As oestrogen levels decrease during menopause, statistics indicate divorce rates increase, and they are initiated by women. This is not just about dissatisfaction with their partners; it often represents a deeper existential questioning of one's place in the world. Menopause is a time when women move away from the traditional norm of self-sacrifice and begin to assert their own identity and desires more strongly. This shift towards self-discovery can be one of the most transformative periods in a woman's life, reshaping her relationships and sense of self.

Rediscovering Yourself

Post menopause is an intriguing phase because it can feel like everything finally calms down. This transition can take up to a decade; like childbirth, it takes time if we allow it to unfold naturally. What's fascinating is that after menopause, our hormone levels often return to the levels they were before menstruation began—the pre-menarche phase before the veil of oestrogen came down. This important insight can help us rediscover our true selves as if we are meeting our former selves again. As a result, you may find yourself reconnecting with passions and interests you had before, such as for example being a vegetarian or an animal rights advocate and tapping back into that untamed version of yourself.

I find the hormonal changes fascinating, especially follicle-stimulating hormone (FSH) and luteinising hormone (LH). These hormones play a crucial role in regulating the menstrual cycle, as they are involved in follicle development and preparing the body for pregnancy. After menopause, FSH and LH levels, which normally fluctuate and peak during ovulation, stabilise at elevated levels similar to those observed during ovulation.

Remember that women often feel their best during ovulation. They tend to feel charismatic, articulate, and attractive during this time. It is interesting to consider the potential effects if these hormone levels remain elevated postmenopausal. Although this has not been extensively studied, there's speculation that sustained high hormone levels might enhance intuition and visionary abilities. These traits seem to flourish in many women after menopause.

Maga, The Wisdom Woman

I first came across the concept of the Maga Wisdom Woman from one of my mentors, Dr Cedar Barstow, who lives in Boulder, Colorado. I was visiting her in my early forties, and she, being about 15 years my senior, introduced me to an incredible, spiritually connected community of women. These women, all about the same age, shared the journey through menopause. With many of their mothers and grandmothers still alive, they knew they were not yet crones, representing the winter of a woman's life. Instead, they were transitioning from summer—the time of being mothers—to the autumn moment of their lives.

The group of friends needed to define this autumn season of their lives, so they chose to call it 'Maga,' drawing from 'magus,' a term used for men in their 50s to 70s known for their wisdom and magical abilities. Thus, 'Maga' became their term, symbolising the female equivalent of a magician. They embraced powerful labels for this stage—empress, enchantress, queen, grandmother, matriarch, and my favourite, 'boss witch.'

Each label reflects this time's unique power, wisdom, and nurturing energy. Embracing these terms gave them a sense of identity and empowered them to navigate this life phase confidently and gracefully. For me, adopting the 'Maga' identity was transformative. It allowed me to reconnect with my inner strength and wisdom and to see this as a time of renewed purpose and self-discovery.

Connecting to Nature

Seeing how many people feel disconnected from nature and view it as something separate from themselves is disheartening. However, it is important to remember that we are not just visitors but integral components of nature. We share the same elements and influences as other animals on this planet.

In our modern world, this disconnect has become a significant issue. I always stress the importance of recognising our inherent connection to nature. Whenever I am puzzled or need clarity, especially when faced with the relentless growth-focused mentality of our capitalist culture, I turn to nature's wisdom. In nature, nothing healthy grows indefinitely without cycling through stages of birth, growth, full bloom, harvest, decay, death, and rebirth. It is a continuous loop; everything in nature undergoes this cycle at different paces.

This process is crucial, and I help women reconnect with it. It is not that we have never been aware of this; rather, we have forgotten. Our society does not embrace these natural processes. The pandemic, for instance, was a stark reminder of this. While not everyone had the opportunity to rest during the pandemic, and many worked harder than ever, it gave us a glimpse of what happens when human activity slows down. We observed the impact of stepping back, even briefly.

This lack of appreciation for the wisdom of cycles is at the heart of many issues. Menstrual pathology, for example, can impact other phases of life; menstrual shame and traumatic childbirth experiences can predispose women to challenging transitions into menopause. Understanding nature puts all these stages into context and reminds us that everything is interconnected. This knowledge used to be more prevalent, but we've gradually lost touch with it over the past centuries.

Herstory

I have written a document called *Herstory*, which is a play on words as opposed to 'his story' or 'history.' It explores how the patriarchy has affected both men and women. I encourage everyone curious about our discussion to read it. The document outlines the characteristics of a patriarchal culture and shows how, as we have become more industrialised, we have started treating everything, including our bodies, like machines. This could not be further from the truth.

Herstory explores important themes such as the historical origins of patriarchy, its influence on gender roles, and how industrialisation has exacerbated these effects. By examining how we have been conditioned to perceive our bodies and identities in a mechanistic way, *Herstory* urges readers to reconsider these ingrained perspectives.

Our Mothers, Ourselves

The experiences of our mothers during their menopause have a significant impact on our own perimenopausal and menopausal journeys. Remarkably, this connection begins even before we're born. During pregnancy, when a woman is carrying a daughter, all the eggs her foetus will ever have are already forming in her ovaries around the 20-week mark into the pregnancy. This means that while your mother was in your grandmother's womb, the egg that would eventually become you was already developing. We were all in our grandmothers' wombs, experiencing the environment and influences of that time. The first half of the pregnancy impacts the gene sequences chosen to become each egg.

We were present in our grandmothers' bodies in early form during the second half of our mothers' pregnancies. We also experienced our mothers' birth, remained in their bodies as eggs until we were ovulated and conceived, and eventually grew in our mothers' wombs until birth. This deep intergenerational connection profoundly shapes us.

The Red Thread

The red thread, or mother line, connects us to our female generational ancestors, forming the ecosystem into which we are born. Our mother's womb is like the garden in which we grow. Everything that has impacted every female in our ancestral line is in our DNA and imprinting experiences from being in our mother's body. When you are pregnant, the baby also feels everything you feel and experience. Therefore, we have experienced all of our mother's life while inside her womb until we were born.

During the early years of our lives, children learn through a process called imprinting, which occurs from in utero until around seven years old. Throughout this time, we unquestioningly accept the behaviours and beliefs of our mother, father, and other dominant adults as the norm. As we grow older, we may reflect on these influences and choose to do things differently. Initially, we are imprinted with their ways, choices, and decisions, which significantly influence us.

As we grow older, we often see our mothers go through menopause. Most women either have no recollection of their mother's menopause or remember her being cranky and stressed. Not much was ever spoken about it. The most significant impact our mothers have on us regarding menopause is how they manage their menstrual cycles.

Menopause is not a singular event; it is the culmination of our lives, shaped by everything that preceded it. Whether we actively support or observe our mother as she goes through this phase, her experiences have an impact on us. This influence may lead us to mirror her behaviour or choose a different path, but the important thing to note is that both generational trauma and strengths are passed down from mother to daughter. Whether we are aware of it or not, everything our mother goes through affects us, and her experience with menopause provides valuable insight.

How Do We Break the Cycle?

It is quite simple. The red thread represents the maternal line, and all it takes is for one of the women to say, **'Whoa, this stops with me.'** She must decide not to pass on the trauma unconsciously. By doing her inner work, she breaks the cycle.

According to the concept of circular time based on Indigenous beliefs, everything happens simultaneously. Therefore, our decisions impact our mothers and grandmothers, as well as our daughters, sons, and grandchildren, even if we never discuss these issues with them. Our inner work influences our behaviour, and it has a ripple effect on future generations. It only takes one person, particularly a woman, to question why they feel a certain way and to seek healing. Healing does not require going back in time; it involves addressing the issues in our lives and breaking the cycle.

By embracing this concept and doing the necessary inner work, we can break the cycle of trauma and create a healthier, more connected future for ourselves and future generations. This transformative journey not only heals us but also honours the women who came before us and those who will come after. Let us be the ones to initiate this change, ensuring a legacy of healing and strength for generations to come.

The Dark Goddess

The Dark Goddess represents our inner voice, guiding us towards necessary change, which we often ignore to our detriment. If we disregard the voice of the inner goddess, we overlook important messages. Whether we refer to it as the dark goddess, the light goddess, or in other ways, it all comes down to the part of ourselves that calls for positive change. You do not have to search for this voice; you are already aware of it. Consider the moments when you have said to yourself, 'I shouldn't have that extra glass of wine,' 'I need to quit smoking,' or 'I really should go for a walk.' If you explore further, you will uncover why you are not hearing these prompts.

In the School of Shamanic Womancraft, we intentionally visit the Dark Goddess to explore inner work and healing. The dark goddess is often found in mythology in the underworld, as seen in stories like The Descent of Inanna, an ancient Sumerian tale, where she visits her sister, Ereshkigal. By re-enacting this myth and deliberately journeying to the underworld, we aim to address our inner struggles and healing needs instead of waiting for life to force us into confronting them through sickness, mental health issues, accidents, or other challenges that arise when we ignore the need to heal or change.

On this meaningful journey to encounter the dark goddess, we discover how we embody different roles in our lives in a wounded manner. We seek guidance from the dark goddess on how to heal. She is not a villain but an ally, leading us towards transformation and healing.

Menopause can feel like a journey into the underworld, recurring and filled with emotional depth. In our culture, there is often a focus on staying in the light and shying away from exploring deeper emotions. Feelings are often labelled as disorders, for example, feeling down might prompt someone to think they have depression, or feeling nervous might lead to thoughts of having anxiety. It is important to recognise that experiencing emotions does not necessarily mean having a specific disorder. While severe mental health conditions are real, there is also a tendency to label regular emotions as problems, which can make people afraid to confront and address them. This fear arises from the association of feeling emotions with having something fundamentally wrong with oneself. Our culture has pathologised feelings.

Understanding why and how you do what you do is important so that you can heal and transform. Instead of acting unconsciously, bring consciousness to your actions. This is a crucial aspect of menopause and any rite of passage. When we reach a rite of passage, the generational trauma we carry as women often surfaces because it is a time of transformation. We come to a fork in the road: we can either continue on the usual path—the way things have always been for me, my family, my community, or our culture—or take a different path. The usual path is often the wounded way, though we might not realise it.

The alternative is to choose the path of healing. To begin this process, you must first acknowledge that you have been on the wounded path and then engage in inner work that bridges the gap between these two paths, guiding you towards healing. While this does not guarantee immediate improvement in everything, it means that you can start becoming aware of the choices and perspectives that will lead you towards the direction you desire.

When we come to menopause, it brings up the same issues that all our previous rites of passage did because one rite of passage leads to the next. The girl who was initiated into womanhood at menarche is the woman who shows up to give birth, already conditioned on how to behave as a woman to be accepted in our culture. You only have to look at the intervention statistics to see how that unfolds. Then comes menopause, the culmination of all that conditioning. With the veil of oestrogen gone, we find ourselves different.

It is like we are undergoing a rebirth, with each change acting as a contraction before we emerge as a new version of ourselves.

Changing Attitudes Towards Menopause

The cultural perspective of society is undergoing a significant shift, largely due to the widespread use of the internet, social media, and the democratisation of information. We now have easy access to research information about drug's side effects, dosages, and more. This level of access is liberating and sheds light on the extent to which information has been kept from us. Late baby boomers and Generation X are now openly discussing menopause, which was once a taboo subject. These open conversations, rare in the past, are the most noticeable change I have observed.

Everything else in terms of attitudes and views on menopause in our culture is predictable. We have learned so much from childbirth, which we need to bring into menopause so we do not have to learn it all over again. But as we know, humans usually do not learn from their mistakes. However, if we take what we have learned from childbirth into menopause, we will see groups of women going in different directions.

When it comes to giving birth, some women choose to take control of their experience by opting for home births or birth centres, while others prefer the care of a specialist obstetrician in a private hospital. The same diversity of choice will likely exist when it comes to menopause. This perspective is not meant to disrespect anyone; it is simply a philosophical view of our bodies, natural processes, and life transitions. In the context of childbirth, there is a difference in philosophy between the approach of a wise woman or midwifery and that of obstetrics. The midwifery approach sees childbirth as a normal, natural process that may sometimes require medical assistance. At the same time, the obstetric perspective views birth as a potentially dangerous process full of risk that needs to be carefully managed.

Applying this to menopause, some women will want to flow with the experience and get the most out of it naturally. There is a big difference in what happens for a woman who has a natural childbirth with no drugs compared to one who has every medical intervention. The same differences will play out in how women approach menopause.

There is a huge difference in what happens for a woman who chooses an unmedicated menopause versus one who chooses a medicated menopause. We have been groomed to medicate our rites of passage: the menstrual cycle, childbirth, menopause, and even death. It is no surprise, but we are already seeing a polarisation of choices, decisions, and philosophies around menopause. Each side often blames the other for being wrong, just like the arguments around childbirth. People say, 'You're wrong; that's dangerous. You have to do it this way.' The same debates are happening with menopause.

There is a growing 16 billion dollar industry encompassing both conventional and alternative forms of hormone replacement therapy (HRT). Since its inception in the 1960s, HRT has undergone significant changes. This leads us to an interesting new topic: the financial aspect and the importance of following the money. Exploring the economic impacts of these changes is intriguing as they mirror broader societal attitudes towards menopause and aging.

As we continue to navigate these choices and debates, it is important to recognise that each woman's journey through menopause is unique. Respecting diverse perspectives and approaches can lead to a more inclusive and supportive dialogue. By understanding and honouring the different ways women experience menopause, we can foster a culture of empathy and empowerment.

Community: The Power of the Circle

One of the most important practices is for women to come together in circles, fostering community and shared wisdom. This practice is not new; it is ancient. When I create women's circles, I often tell women that if this is their first circle and it feels vaguely familiar, it is because we have been sitting in circles longer than we have not. It is a recreation of the village and the community we all long for.

In women's circles, we can educate each other about what it means to be a woman, including topics like the menstrual cycle, childbirth, and menopause. We can support each other when we are all on the same page. In a healing women's circle, which must be a safe place, we establish conditions such as confidentiality, non-judgment, and not giving advice—just listening and supporting each other. The magic that happens in these circles is incredible. When we are alone, we tell ourselves stories about how bad things are, how we will not survive, or how inconvenient everything is. But in a circle, we realise we are not alone. We might hear, 'Oh my God, she's experiencing that too. I thought I was the only one.' That connection, commonality, and sisterhood are what we need.

Women naturally have a unique way of dealing with stress, known as 'tend and befriend,' in addition to fight-or-flight. This process involves women coming together, supporting, and caring for each other and their children. Studying the 'tend and befriend' phenomenon is important because it is how we operate under stress and is essential for our wellbeing.

Our natural biological tendency is to gather and support one another purposefully. In the United Kingdom, this approach is known as community prescribing, and the NHS is embracing it because it is low-cost and has no physical side effects. Creating connections and coming together is similar to forming a women's circle, which serves as the heart and hearth of a community or village. We all need this sense of community. COVID has shown us the importance of community, particularly when dealing with isolation.

Creating a women's circle helps form the village. I always suggest this to women at various stages of their lives, especially when they have young children. Finding your women's circle is ideal, as it will serve as the village where you celebrate your rites of passage together. Our rites of passage are community and cultural events, which makes them so significant. Whatever happens during a rite of passage, such as menopause, teaches us how our culture values the next role we are going into—the Wise Women.

Our culture teaches us not to value certain things. Instead of focusing on youth, beauty, and sexual availability, we should realise that change is inevitable. Nature does not allow us to stay in any place forever. Life evolves, and we need to adapt accordingly.

The Wisdom of Post-Menopausal Women

Humanity is currently experiencing a phase similar to perimenopause, and women's wisdom is critical to our evolution. The fact that human women live past their reproductive years has baffled evolutionary biologists. They have researched other animals that go through menopause, including pilot whales, orcas, beluga whales, and narwhals. Their research has revealed that post reproductive grandmother whales in these species serve as leaders of their group/pods. This suggests that the purpose of menopause in these mammals is related to leadership.

As we experience these periods of change, it is important to acknowledge and respect the wisdom and leadership that come with age and experience. By coming together and engaging in women's circle gatherings, we can build supportive communities that celebrate every stage of life. This can help foster a culture of empathy, empowerment, and growth.

Doing the Inner Work

What I suggest for women going through perimenopause or menopause is to do their inner work. The simplest message is, to be with what is—not what you wish was happening or not happening but be present with your current experience. Whether it is a hot flush, insomnia, vaginal dryness, or sexual issues, ask yourself:

How does this serve my transformation? That is what is happening: transformation, not just symptoms.

For example, it took me eight years to realise that when I was experiencing hot flushes, I never took off my jumper; instead, I would breathe through it and endure the discomfort. When I finally noticed what I was doing—after eight years—it unravelled my whole life. I realised I had been enduring so many things throughout my life. I traced it back to its origin when I was a child, quite sick, and had to endure many things. It was an ingrained way of managing. So, it is not the symptom that gives us the message; it is our reaction. It is what arises for us in response.

In my journey dealing with changes in my libido and sexuality, I rediscovered my inner maiden and all that she contributed to my sexual identity. I realised that I needed to heal her to progress as a sexual being in my postmenopausal years. This was something I had not realised I needed to do. So, it is about accepting the present, observing what comes up, and using those experiences as steps towards becoming a healed version of yourself.

I have noticed from personal experience and from listening to many women in similar situations that a lot of the inner work during menopause is related to inner child work. It involves healing childhood trauma. We understand that one rite of passage leads to the next, so it is important to delve into your past. Become a bit of a forensic archaeologist in your life and discover all the generational trauma you have inherited. You may be unconscious of it, but being aware is crucial. Look into your mother's and grandmother's lives to understand what female red thread you have inherited.

It is important to understand the circumstances of your birth and its impact on your life. Instead of being controlled by it, learn to work with it. Reflect on your first menstruation experience and the societal expectations it brought. Recognise your internalised negative beliefs and replace them with positive, empowering messages. Train your brain to embrace positive ideas about womanhood, as these beliefs may not have been instilled in you as a child. Remember, our brains are adaptable, so you can shift your perspective by consistently reinforcing positive messages.

Your first sexual experience impacts how you transform sexually at menopause. Everyone has a big story about this, one way or another. Sometimes, it is abuse or nonconsensual experiences. Sexual healing is possible at menopause if you explore deeply and have support.

Consider all the pregnancies you have experienced. Each pregnancy leads to some form of birth, whether it is a loss or an abortion. Reflecting on all your pregnancies and births to learn from them is critical to becoming a wise woman. Focusing on the positive lessons from these experiences, rather than just the hardships, is important.

The Birthing Formula refers to the chronological teachings of the womb, which prepare each woman for menopause. Similarly, the teachings of menopause are preparation for death, although I cannot confirm that personally.

Embracing these insights and doing the inner work can lead to personal transformation. By understanding and healing from our past, we can navigate menopause and other life transitions with greater awareness and strength.

What Brings Me Joy

At this moment, my grandchildren fill me with joy. Their presence motivates me to stay fit and strong, mainly so I can lift them. This drive comes from understanding how our sedentary lifestyles and lack of functional exercise contribute to weaker bones. Weight-bearing exercises send our bones the message through our muscles that they need to stay strong. So, carrying my grandchildren not only brings me joy but also helps build stronger bones.

Another source of joy is witnessing women awakening to their inherent power. It is exhilarating to see women emerge from the shadows of patriarchal influence, embracing their autonomy, sovereignty, and the full breadth of their capabilities. This collective awakening signifies a crucial evolution, promising great impacts across all aspects of life.

Where to Find Out More About Jane Hardwicke Collings

To delve deeper into the wisdom shared by Jane Hardwicke Collings, visit her School of Shamanic Womancraft at schoolofshamanicwomancraft.com. This school offers courses, workshops, and resources that empower women to reconnect with the wisdom of the cycles and embrace their own transformative journeys.

Jane's upcoming book, Sagescence, explores menopause as a rite of passage similar to adolescence and matrescence. She introduces Sagescence as the journey to becoming a wise woman, focusing on transformation beyond just the physical aspects. Through *Sagescence*, Jane invites readers to embrace this term and dive into the wisdom it holds.

In addition to her upcoming book, Jane offers *Altar Cards* that teach the wisdom of the cycle, a cycle-tracking app, and a variety of courses that help women align with their natural rhythms. Her website provides more information on these offerings, allowing women to fully participate in this meaningful journey of self-discovery and empowerment.

Final Thoughts

I am thrilled to share this journey with you. I hope my books and tools inspire and empower you to embrace your natural rhythms and step into your full potential. Your participation in this journey is what makes it truly meaningful.

The evolution we are experiencing as women is not just personal; it is a significant cultural shift affecting all areas of life. Let us embrace it together.

Reflection on My Conversation with Jane

After my conversation with Jane Hardwicke Collings, I was in awe of her wisdom. Although I had encountered Jane's insights through podcasts and books, hearing them directly from her added a new depth. The strength and 'boss witch' energy she exuded transcended the digital barrier of our laptop screens. I felt a tinge of sadness for not discovering her work earlier, particularly during my transition into motherhood. I wonder how different my approach to that phase of my life might have been.

Realising My Own Institutionalised Abuse During Childbirth

This conversation with Jane made it clear that I had also been a victim of institutionalised abuse disguised as safety measures, especially during the birth of my first child. My experience underscores many important issues Jane highlighted and emphasises the need for greater awareness and advocacy for respectful and supportive birthing practices.

In 2008, far from my family, I decided to go to a private hospital for my delivery. I did not know what to expect. My obstetrician strongly recommended scheduling a caesarean section, but I was determined to have a natural birth. When that seemed impossible, she convinced me to be induced at 38 weeks—a decision I have regretted ever since. My obstetrician appeared sporadically during labour, making brief appearances between other births or appointments. The hours dragged on. After more than 10 hours of labour, as I neared my breaking point, she began persuading my husband to agree to an epidural. Seeing my exhaustion, he reluctantly consented. The transformation in the labour ward was immediate and shocking, with nurses, an anaesthetist, and doctors swiftly gathering for the procedure. Fortunately, a midwife intervened, suggesting one more check to see how far I was dilated. She gently examined me and smiled, 'You're already 8 cm. It is too late for the epidural.' Relief washed over me, but it was short-lived. Despite this, my obstetrician escalated the intervention by performing an episiotomy, cutting me even though I felt confident I could have delivered my tiny, 2.3-kilogram baby naturally.

After the birth, the overwhelming love for my baby took over, pushing this experience to the back of my mind as the joy and connection with my newborn consumed me.

Later, I discovered that private hospitals profited more from caesarean sections and epidurals. This revelation deepened my sense of violation, as it became clear that financial incentives often outweighed the well-being of birthing women. This experience took away my ability to fully engage in natural birthing. More importantly, it altered my daughter's entrance into the world, with potential lifelong effects. At the time, I did not fully understand the extent of what was taken from me. Looking back, it is clear that this was a stark example of how institutional protocols and the over-medicalisation of childbirth can strip away a woman's autonomy and empowerment.

A Different Experience with My Second Daughter

In 2012, I welcomed my second daughter into the world at a public hospital without an assigned obstetrician or the pressure to schedule a caesarean. At 38 weeks, I was once again induced. The kind midwife guided me through each contraction, encouraging me to envision them as waves in the ocean. This visualisation helped me manage the pain and feel deeply connected to nature, even within the sterile surroundings. During labour, I felt transported to another dimension. My heart swelled with immense love as I gave birth to my second daughter. This moment was the essence of human existence, a powerful act of bringing new life into the world. In that instant, I glimpsed the life force guiding me, with the midwife appearing as a beautiful, angelic presence. She transformed the clinical atmosphere into connection and love, creating a natural environment through visualisation amidst the hospital's sterility.

Reflecting on these experiences, I realise the impact of institutionalised birthing practices and the crucial role of supportive, empowering care. My journey emphasises the importance of advocating for women's autonomy and respectful treatment during childbirth.

Although at times painful, the experiences highlight the significance of Jane's work and the need for ongoing discussions to improve women's birthing experiences. They also emphasise the importance of taking ownership of my own rites of passage. As I approach menopause, I was determined to navigate this transition on my own terms, ensuring that it is respected and honoured as a natural and empowering process. Understanding these dynamics has strengthened my commitment to advocating for women's autonomy and empowerment during all significant life transitions.

Hygieia Health: A Mission Born from Crisis

Jane is not only a revered leader in women's spiritual health and wisdom but also one of the co-founders of Hygieia Health, a not-for-profit charity dedicated to raising awareness about birth trauma and providing healing solutions and preventative measures.

Hygeia Health started in 2020, just as COVID-19 began to spread globally. Recognising the urgent need for support, Hygieia Health established a Facebook group called 'Mamatoto' in Swahili; this means 'Motherbaby,' reflecting the idea that mother and baby are one interrelated entity; what affects one affects the other. This online forum quickly became a sanctuary for mothers, fathers, midwives, and doulas to come together and navigate the unexpected and tumultuous time affecting everyone, especially pregnant and birthing mothers.

Discovering 'Herstory'

After our discussion, I downloaded Jane's book *Herstory.* It's a short but impactful narrative about an ancient matriarchal society that worshipped the goddess and valued Mother Nature. Here is a brief summary:

Around 40,000 years ago, women played significant roles in society, as evidenced by cave paintings and carvings. However, around 3000 BC, patriarchal tribes took over, leading to a decline in women's status and property rights. Female healers were persecuted and killed during the Inquisition. Despite these difficulties, 'Herstory' shows resilience. Today, there is a renewed respect for women's wisdom and nature, leading to a revival of feminine power.

This narrative emphasises the enduring strength and resilience of women throughout history. The resurgence of feminine power today is a testament to the importance of reconnecting with our roots and embracing the wisdom passed down through generations.

Looking Forward

I am grateful that we have moved beyond those dark times in history. Had we lived in those eras, we might have been killed or burned simply for sharing these stories—just like the millions of women who suffered such fates.

Postmenopausal women possess immense power, and it is no wonder the patriarchy has historically worked to silence them. In the past, postmenopausal women were often the intuitive visionaries who led their communities with compassion and wisdom. They were the 'wise women' who held roles of guidance and healing—until they were persecuted. This history speaks to our enormous potential to create positive change.

Now, it is time for postmenopausal women to rise and reclaim our place in our communities, contributing in whatever ways we can to help future generations live fulfilling lives without fear of societal persecution. We must share our gifts and knowledge, drawing from our experiences to uplift and empower those around us.

As we move forward, let us embrace the power and wisdom that come with age. By using our voices and experiences, we can foster a culture of empathy, empowerment, and growth. In doing so, we ensure that future generations benefit from the hard-earned wisdom of their elders, living in a world that values and respects the contributions of all its members.

Reflection Activity:
Embracing Your Inner Journey

This activity sheet is designed to guide you through a journey of self-discovery inspired by insights from Jane Hardwicke Collings. Reflect on your experiences, honour your personal path, and work towards becoming a more healed version of yourself. By examining your family history, monitoring your emotions, and connecting with your inner self, you will gain valuable insights and develop greater awareness and strength to navigate this phase of life.

Tips for Using These Activities

Emotional Support: If you encounter difficult emotions, consider seeking support from a trusted friend, family member, or professional.

Self-Compassion: Approach these reflections with self-compassion and patience. Be gentle with yourself as you explore these deep aspects of your life.

Pacing and Flexibility: Take your time. There is no rush. Revisit any section as needed and move at your own pace.

Activity 1: Explore Your Family History

Mother's Experience: Write down any stories or observations about how your mother managed menstruation and menopause.

- Consider her emotions and physical experiences. What did she share with you, and what did you observe?

Prompt: 'My mother experienced...'

Grandmother's Experience: Find out what your grandmother experienced while pregnant with your mother. Gather any information from family stories or historical context and write it down.

Prompt: 'During my grandmother's pregnancy with my mother, she...'

Reflection Questions:

- What significant events were happening in your mother's and grandmother's lives during these periods?

- How might their environments and relationships have influenced their experiences?

- How do you think their experiences during these times might have affected you?

Activity 2: Track Your Emotions

Diary: For two weeks, keep a diary of your emotions and physical sensations before a hot flush.

Note the time, your activities, and your thoughts.

Prompt: 'Today, before my hot flush, I felt...'

Reflect:

- Look for patterns in your diary. Are specific thoughts or situations triggering your hot flushes?

- How do stress, anxiety, or other emotions correlate with your symptoms?

- What strategies can you use to manage these emotions and potentially reduce the frequency or intensity of hot flushes?

Activity 3. Tapping into the Aura of the Hot Flush

Observe: Pay attention to physical sensations, emotions, or thoughts before a hot flush starts.

Prompt: 'Before my hot flush, I noticed...'

Write: Document these experiences. Reflect on what these sensations might be communicating about your current state.

Activity 4: Revisiting Your Pre-menarche Self

Remember: Think back to who you were before your first period. What were your hobbies, passions, and dreams?

Prompt: 'As a child, I loved to...'

Reconnect: Write down any interests from that time that still call to you.

- Are there any hobbies or passions you want to revisit?

Activity 5: Connecting with Your Inner Dark Goddess

Inner Dialogue: Set aside weekly time to connect with your inner Dark Goddess, the part of you that demands change and growth.

Prompt: 'My inner Dark Goddess is telling me that I need to...'

Reflect:

- Write down any insights or messages you receive.

- What areas of your life need attention?

- What inner work should you do?

Activity 6: Identifying Patterns and Themes

Identify Patterns: Look for recurring themes or patterns in your family history and personal experiences.

Prompt: 'I noticed a pattern in my family where...'

Reflect:

- Consider how these patterns have impacted different generations in your family.

- What changes would you like to make in your own life and for future generations?

Activity 7: Final Reflection

Look Back: Reflect on the overall process. How has looking back helped you understand your journey better?

Prompt: 'What was the most surprising thing I learned?'

Plan Forward: Write a final reflection on how you plan to move forward with this new awareness. Consider specific actions to integrate these insights into your daily life.

Prompt: 'How will I integrate this new awareness into my daily life?'

Concluding Thoughts

Reflecting on these questions and keeping a diary can help you gain a deeper understanding of your personal history and the patterns that influence your life. Embracing this awareness is a step towards reclaiming your autonomy and empowering yourself in life's transitions. Share your reflections with a trusted friend, family member, or support group to further enhance your understanding and support each other on this journey.

Dr Christiane Northrup

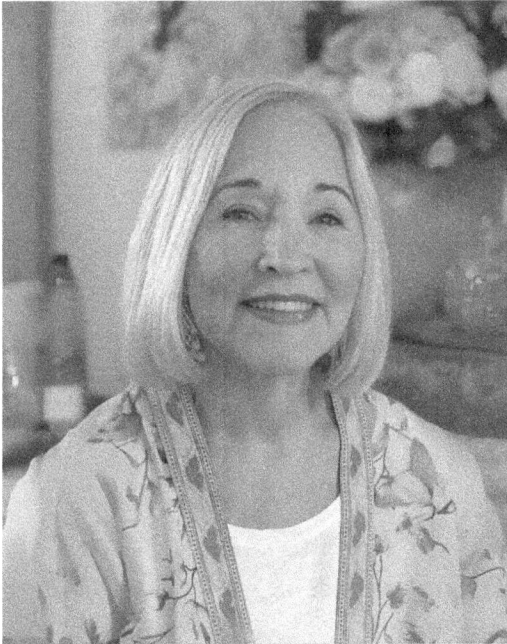

The Ageless Goddess

Discovering Dr Christiane Northrup

In 2015, the first symptoms of perimenopause marked the beginning of a transformative journey for me, leading to an awakening. My body and mind started to communicate with me in new ways: experiencing hot flushes, anxiety, craving junk food, coming to terms with aging in a youth-driven world, and trying to keep up with my old self while a new version of me was trying to be born. The more I tried to cling to the old, the louder my symptoms became until I had to do something radical.

I signed up for a five-day fasting retreat in Byron Bay, and the lovely Sarah Foley from White Lotus Cleansing Retreats looked after me. Even though I had two young children and was on a tight budget, I knew I needed to prioritise some time for myself. I needed space to listen to my inner voice, figure out who I was becoming, and move forward in my life. My old ways of coping were no longer working for me, and the manageable anxiety I once had begun to affect my everyday life, causing stress.

Initially, I sought advice from women who were further along in their menopause journey. However, their whispered accounts of shame and invisibility left me disheartened. I refused to accept the narrative of decline. Deep down, I knew that my life was not over. I sensed that hidden in a corner of my soul was the belief that once I did the inner work, my life was beginning. I did not want to settle into invisibility or succumb to the negative programming surrounding menopause. I was determined to find a different experience and celebrate this transition as a time of growth and wisdom.

The Mother of All Wake-Up Calls

During my fasting retreat, I came across Dr. Christiane Northrup on a wellness show. Her perspective on menopause planted the seed to a new beginning. I recall her words, which have been implanted in my memory ever since: **'Menopause is the mother of all wake-up calls, and it's a time in a woman's life when she becomes who she is meant to be and shouts it out aloud, unapologetically,'** This change in perspective transformed my view of menopause from a time of loss to a powerful new beginning.

Dr Northrup's words not only changed my perspective but also inspired me to document and share my journey, which led to the creation of this book. Taking a leap of faith, I emailed Dr. Northrup on December 28, 2023, outlining my vision and her work's impact on me. To my surprise and delight, her assistant replied positively on January 10, 2024, agreeing to be interviewed. This moment confirmed my path and gave me the confidence to move forward as she was the first wonder of menopause I asked and the first to say yes.

Anticipating Meeting Dr Christiane Northrup

The night before my interview with Dr. Christiane Northrup, I was so excited that I could hardly sleep. The interview was scheduled for 6:30 am, and I was up and ready well before then, eager to speak with someone who had reshaped my understanding of womanhood and my menopause journey.

As I sat in my office, waiting for her to join the Zoom meeting, I didn't expect to be hit with such a wave of emotion. When Dr. Northrup appeared on the screen, tears started flowing down my face as I was grateful for this incredible opportunity. I tried to pull myself together, but the emotions were too powerful. In her usual kind and understanding way, Dr. Northrup gave me a moment to gather myself before we began our conversation. Even though I had prepared extensively, I realised I needed to let go and let the conversation unfold naturally.

Dr. Northrup has helped me understand and manage my perimenopause journey. Her advice was crucial in dealing with physical symptoms. She also helped me see the excitement and new possibilities during this transformative time. Her wisdom deepened my understanding of this stage of life and helped me rediscover and appreciate myself and the deep inner work awaiting me spiritually and physically.

Her support was essential in bringing our book, *Seven Wonders of Menopause,* to life. She was the first to say yes to the project, which inspired me and paved the way for other incredible women to join in. Their trust in me and their willingness to share their stories made this book possible.

I can't express enough gratitude to Dr. Christiane Northrup. Her guidance and encouragement have been the foundation of this journey. I wouldn't have had the courage to take on this project without her. Thank you, Dr. Northrup, for your inspiration and support and for helping bring together the incredible women featured in *Seven Wonders of Menopause*.

Introduction to Dr. Christiane Northrup

Dr. Christiane Northrup is a board-certified Obstetrician-Gynaecologist (OB/GYN) and a pioneer in women's health. Her groundbreaking work has earned her a place on the New York Times bestseller list with influential books such as *Women's Bodies, Women's Wisdom*, *The Wisdom of Menopause*, *Goddesses Never Age*, and *Dodging Energy Vampires*. Dr. Northrup's innovative approach to women's health and wellness has gained widespread recognition.

Dr. Northrup has appeared on The Oprah Winfrey Show ten times and is celebrated as one of Oprah's Super Soul 100, a group of awakened leaders using their voices and talent to elevate humanity. In 2020, 2021, and again in 2022, Watkins Magazine named Dr. Northrup on their 'Watkins Spiritual 100 List' as one of their 100 Most

Spiritually Influential Living People. This list includes spiritual teachers, activists, authors, and thinkers who are changing the world.

Dr. Northrup is a graduate of Dartmouth Medical School and has previously served as a clinical professor of OB/GYN at the University of Vermont College of Medicine. She highlights the intrinsic wisdom of the female body and calls for a more empathetic, personalised approach to women's health that transcends the traditional disease-oriented model.

Dr. Northrup is an author and an engaging speaker who has appeared on various TV programs, including The Dr. Oz Show and Good Morning America. Her influence goes beyond her books and television appearances, as she shares her wisdom through podcasts, online courses, and social media platforms, inspiring and educating a broad audience.

Her outstanding contributions to women's health have earned her numerous awards and honours, including the Reader's Choice Award from The Times of London and the prestigious 2007 International Health & Medical Media Award for her television special, Menopause and Beyond. Dr. Northrup's work focuses on promoting wellness and vitality for women rather than just treating illness, and her holistic approach has redefined the concept of a healthy, vibrant woman in today's world.

In December 2022, the Zelenko Foundation awarded Dr. Northrup the Rosa Parks Fearless Stand for Medical Freedom Award, recognising her dedication to medical freedom. Her advocacy goes beyond her literary works and television appearances, as she urges individuals to trust their instincts and make informed health decisions.

"Menopause is the mother of all wake-up calls.

It's not just about physical symptoms; it's an opportunity to transform and improve your life, and ultimately, our culture."

Dr Christiane Northrup

A Conversation with
Dr. Christiane Northrup

Medical Freedom Rose Parks Award

In December 2022, I was honoured to receive the Rosa Parks Fearless Stand for Medical Freedom Award from the Zelenko Foundation. I remember the moment in Grand Rapids, Michigan, when Kevin Jenkins and I walked by a statue of Rosa Parks. Inspired by her legacy, Kevin decided to recognise those of us who had been tirelessly advocating for medical freedom for decades.

(Rosa Parks was an inspirational figure in the Civil Rights Movement. She is best known for her courageous refusal to give up her bus seat to a white passenger in 1955 in Montgomery, Alabama. Her defiance sparked the Montgomery Bus Boycott and became a powerful symbol of the fight against racial segregation and injustice. The Rosa Parks Award honours individuals who embody their spirit of courage and commitment to justice.)

The ceremony brought together esteemed advocates such as Sherri Tenpenny, Barbara Loe Fisher, and Maura McDonnell. Being in their company and acknowledged for our long-standing efforts was gratifying. This recognition, symbolised by the Rosa Parks Award, is highly significant as it not only honours our past efforts but also fuels my motivation to continue advocating for medical freedom and justice.

Creating a New Language
for Women's Health

When I wrote *Women's Bodies, Women's Wisdom*, I realised I had to create a new language for women's health, not women's diseases. Here's what I learned: the way women's health is practised often sends the message, 'You don't have it yet, but keep coming back because we have better and better tests to determine what is wrong, and sooner or later, we will find it.' This approach suggests that there is always something wrong waiting to be discovered.

Instead of affirming that 'you're doing beautifully, continue,' the system produces increasingly sophisticated tests to find ever smaller issues, leading to drastic measures like removing breasts and uteruses, making women feel bad about themselves.

My Menopause Journey
and Appearing on Oprah

When I was going through menopause, it was a difficult and transformative time for me. I've detailed my experience in my book, but to give a short summary, I was also going through a divorce, which began the day after my first appearance on Oprah.

Let me share with you what happened. I was on Oprah, and at that time, they filmed the B-roll in Chicago. I went through all that, and then, a week later, the show aired. I sat down at 4 p.m., excited to watch my big moment on Oprah. However, my youngest daughter was more interested in playing with her friends and did not want to watch. Meanwhile, my then-husband wanted me to look at something with his ear and kept taking phone calls.

While my office phone rang off the hook, people congratulated me and said how wonderful it was. In my own home, I got no recognition except from my oldest daughter. There was no celebration, no acknowledgment of my achievement. This was a symbolic story of my experience at that time. Although things have changed now, it was clear to me what was happening back then.

My appearance on Oprah, which should have been a celebratory milestone, was overshadowed by the lack of recognition and support from those closest to me.

Breaking out of Traditional Moulds

I was one of the first women to break away from traditional roles. There were always some women who were doctors, but they were rare. Then, in the 1970s, many more of us became lawyers, doctors, and other professionals.

It was a time when my mother could not even get a loan in her own name after my dad died, but things started to change. However, I still had the mindset of the 1950s: I just wanted to be married, to be Mrs. So-and-So, and to treat my career as a hobby so I would not cause any trouble.

I didn't realise it then, but I knew how to stay married and keep my husband happy. Another part of me understood that everything starts with consciousness. I had worked with the medical intuitive Caroline Myss. She taught me that our consciousness shapes our bodies and lives.

I felt torn between two distinct parts of my life. On the outside, I was making a global impact on women's health, but inside, I was trying to meet societal expectations. These conflicting parts of my life eventually collided.

I realised that if I continued this way, I would develop bilateral inflammatory breast cancer and risk dying within three years. I had seen this pattern before, and Caroline Myss even told me that cancer viruses had been in and out of my body since I was in my thirties. She warned me that if I had not left my practice and moved, I would have developed a large ovarian cyst since ovaries symbolise ambition. **We often say a man has 'balls' while a woman has 'ovaries.'**

Embracing Our True Selves

In my personal life, I realised that I had been pretending not to be the influential change-maker I truly was. This internal conflict was unsustainable, and it could have serious health consequences if I did not live authentically. This journey taught me that acknowledging and integrating our ambitions and true selves into our lives is important. Trying to conform to traditional roles or suppress our true nature can have severe physical and emotional consequences. Embracing our true selves and living authentically is crucial for our well-being and fulfilment.

It was about pushing for what I wanted to see happen, but it becomes unhealthy when you push your own agency through a husband, a grant, or any external validation. We all have lessons about how we are meant to co-create with divinity, with our true selves. I kept waiting for the powers above to accept my ideas, but they did not. I did not want to make them wrong because I loved my profession and the best aspects of Western medicine. I realised that I would have to figure this out on my own.

Walking through a Wall of Fire

When I first wrote *Women's Bodies, Women's Wisdom*, the very first edition, I would wake up every night thinking someone was in the house trying to kill me.

Rupert Sheldrake, a British biologist, talks about the presence of the past or the morphogenic field. **Those who do anything outside the norm often have to walk through a wall of fire**, reminiscent of the burning times when nine million women—healers, midwives, herbalists—were burned as witches. Entire towns in Germany during the Middle Ages were left without a single girl or woman. The feminine has been under attack on planet Earth for about 6,000 years.

Think about that for a moment. The fear and oppression of feminine energy have deep roots in our collective history.

Mother of Power

I realised that in every place where women's power exists, we've been taught to fear and deny it. For instance, consider the mother of power in ancient cultures, **where women who retained their sacred blood could lead their communities**. It's no coincidence that post-menopausal women often become shamans and community leaders. While there are powerful women before menopause, they truly come into their own after menopause when their brains change.

Once menopause is reached, the levels of Follicle-Stimulating Hormone (FSH) and Luteinising Hormone (LH) remain at ovulatory levels for the rest of your life. This allows you to see connections that others may not recognise. However, society often portrays menopause as the end of femininity, sexuality, and attractiveness. Mainstream movies even suggest that it's more likely for a woman over 40 to be killed by a terrorist than to get married.

Challenging and overturning cultural myths and negative stereotypes has always been my aim. I strongly believe that our focus and beliefs shape our reality. Menopause is often viewed as a decline in a woman's life, but I see it as the beginning of true wisdom, mastery, and an enjoyable chapter of life. I hope that you too can see it that way too.

Goddesses Never Age

I wanted to share this meaningful quote from my colleague Dr. Mario Martinez, who wrote *The MindBody Code* and played a significant role in my research for *Goddesses Never Age*. Dr. Martinez once said, **'Getting older is inevitable, aging is optional,' or 'Getting older is the opportunity to increase your value and competence.'** This phrase resonated with me, and I made it my truth. When I wrote *Goddesses Never Age*, I was determined to explore whether society's belief that a woman's attractiveness diminishes with age was true or just a cultural myth.

What I discovered was exhilarating. More comes by being open to more life, joy, and experiences. My postmenopausal life has been more fun and more fulfilling than ever before. So, welcome this transition. Your journey is just beginning, and it is more beautiful than you have been led to believe.

Before appearing on Oprah, I faced various challenges, including navigating through multiple lawsuits, which is a common experience for many OB/GYNs. Unfortunately, our culture often promotes suing doctors when outcomes aren't perfect instead of emphasising personal responsibility for one's own health.

I have faced many fires of transformation, each one refining me to turning iron into steel. So, when March of 2020 hit and I knew something was way off, I couldn't keep my mouth shut.

Dealing with Loss

The transition to perimenopause is a period of physical, emotional, and spiritual change. How do we move through these shifts? It involves a holistic approach, acknowledging and embracing the changes occurring on every level of your being, and learning to navigate this new phase with grace and understanding.

Firstly, it is essential to acknowledge that growth often comes hand-in-hand with loss. This is a fundamental part of life.

When you have a baby, for example, you lose your maidenhood and a great deal of your freedom. When my first baby was born, I was on the porch of my house preparing to go grocery shopping. For a brief moment, I forgot I had a baby and was going to get in the car and go. It suddenly hit me, 'Oh my gosh, you have ruined your life.' That feeling was fleeting but significant, marking the loss of my former freedom.

Entering the Wisdom Years

As you enter Perimenopause, it is a significant and often challenging transition that can last for several years, ranging from 6 to 13 years. During this time, women move from the cyclical wisdom of menstruation, with its peaks in hormones like FSH and LH during ovulation and high testosterone levels, to a different kind of wisdom in the later years.

However, for many women, it can be abrupt, especially if they undergo procedures such as a hysterectomy with ovary removal, which instantly brings about changes in their brain, a phase often referred to as their 'wisdom years.'

During this time, emotions can run high, and society often uses this against women. Anger during menopause is frequently a result of having 'de-selfed' oneself to be acceptable to others. I remember my own mother's frustration during menopause, the desire to throw the roast out of the window, a metaphor for the deeper discontent brewing inside. The beauty of reaching the other end of menopause is the realisation that giving away your essence to please others removes you from genuine relationships.

On a broader scale, consider what's happening on the planet: We're often not allowed to express certain opinions or truths, which prevents genuine relationships.

After menopause, speaking your truth becomes a form of self-care. However, it's not about splattering it all over everyone or pointing out others' wrongs. It's about softening, coming home to your heart, and healing the wounds of your inner child.

Adolescence in Reverse

Perimenopause is like adolescence in reverse, a time to reconcile with parts of yourself that may have been neglected or suppressed, ultimately allowing you to emerge wiser and more authentic.

I emphasised, delving deeper into the transformative journey of perimenopause. Think back to when you were around 11 or 12 years old. You had a clearer sense of who you were and what you loved before the hormonal shifts of puberty. As oestrogen levels begin to rise, that clarity can become clouded, and suddenly, external forces attempt to define you. Your menstrual cycle may become erratic, but you find your footing again by your twenties.

As you enter perimenopause, you may find yourself rediscovering your true self. Women need to realise that if they stay healthy, their post-menopausal years can last just as long as their reproductive years. So, you do not lose anything significant. While you may lose the ability to have a child biologically, you gain so much more.

There is a period of grief if you have waited until 48 to have children and find it is too late. But even then, I have known women who have had children naturally at that age, demonstrating the wonders of the female body, which we do not fully appreciate.

Cultural Believes

While serving as the American Holistic Medical Association president, I met a shaman named Brant Secunda. Brant became a shaman with the Huichol tribe in northern Mexico after originally travelling from Queens, New York. During our conversation, Brant shared that the Huichol tribe held a belief that a baby was a divine gift and that women in the tribe had babies well into their 50s and 60s. This challenged the notion that their eggs were too old for conception and served as a powerful example of how cultural beliefs can significantly impact our biology.

For example, a woman in her forties may visit her doctor and be advised to get a mammogram, flu shot, or pneumovax and to start considering colonoscopies. If she declines, the doctor may express concern, citing statistics that show health tends to decline after 50. However, this decline is often a result of not taking care of oneself over the years. Perimenopause serves as a wake-up call, indicating that continuing old habits can lead to higher risks of breast cancer, high blood pressure, and other health conditions.

In the United States, the average 65-year-old is on seven prescription drugs. This is not inevitable. Perimenopause can be a time to reassess and make changes that improve your health and well-being rather than accepting a decline. It's about coming home to your heart, recognising and healing past wounds, and embracing this phase as an opportunity for growth and renewal.

The journey through perimenopause and beyond is about reclaiming your power and wisdom. It's a time to honour your body's signals, nurture your emotional well-being, and connect with your spiritual essence. Doing so can transform this phase into one of your life's most empowering and fulfilling periods.

HRT and its Introduction

I remember seeing *Feminine Forever* by Robert A. Wilson in the medical library when I was a medical student in Plainfield Vermont. The book advocated for Hormone Replacement Therapy (HRT) and discussed Premarin, an oestrogen medication derived from pregnant horse urine. At that time, oestrogen was primarily obtained from pregnant horse urine because they hadn't yet developed a method to synthesize it from wild Mexican yams or soybeans. It's important to note that this type of oestrogen is not recommended, and there are better options available.

The backstory is quite intriguing: During perimenopause, Robert Wilson's wife started asserting herself. The concept of *Feminine Forever* implied 'missive forever.' When his wife ceased to be a pushover, Wilson attributed this change to menopause instead of recognising it as a positive transformation.

(Hormone Replacement Therapy (HRT) was introduced in the 1940s and gained mainstream attention in the 1960s, particularly after Dr. Robert Wilson's 1966 book Feminine Forever promoted oestrogen therapy as a way to preserve youthfulness in menopausal women (Wilson, 1966). By the 1970s and 1980s, HRT usage increased with the introduction of combined HRT, which reduced the risk of endometrial cancer (Utian, 1975). The therapy became widely prescribed in the 1990s, not only for managing menopausal symptoms but also for its believed benefits in preventing osteoporosis and heart disease.

However, the 2002 Women's Health Initiative (WHI) study raised concerns about the risks of HRT, such as increased chances of breast cancer, heart disease, and stroke, leading to a decline in its use (Rossouw et al., 2002). Since then, HRT has been approached more cautiously, with individualised assessments of its risks and benefits for each woman.)

The Crossover

When I appeared on Oprah with *The Wisdom of Menopause* in 2001, it was groundbreaking. She had men on the show because my working premise, which is true, is that a woman is often deeply involved in her family's inner world. As she enters menopause, she often feels a desire to go out into the world. Conversely, many men at this stage of life start wanting to come back into the home. There is this crossover, and I encouraged men to support their wives during this time. It is her turn to venture into the world.

The B-roll footage from that show was excellent. We featured women who had started businesses, such as a quilt company. Their husbands discussed how their marriages were better than ever. It is important to take care of yourself during perimenopause, as you may be at risk of developing chronic illnesses. Lewis Thomas, the former head of Memorial Sloan Kettering Cancer, once said, 'I've come to believe that cancer is the physical metaphor for the extreme need to grow.'

What Should You Do During Perimenopause?

Start by examining the health history of your mother, her sisters, and other female relatives. What illnesses run in your family? Then, go deeper and ask yourself about the emotional patterns, belief systems, and behaviours that run in your family.

For instance, I have a friend who observed that all of her mother's sisters, as well as her mother herself, gained weight, started wearing muumuus, and spent their days watching soap operas. She decided she was not going to follow that pattern. She took action to avoid chronic arthritis, Graves' disease, and other ailments. She said, 'I don't have those issues because I decided I'm not doing this.

When certain traits or conditions appear to be passed from one generation to the next, it's important to understand that your genes and your DNA do not predetermine your future. In his book *The Biology of Belief*, Bruce Lipton explains this concept well. He states that the cell membrane, acting as the cell's brain, constantly responds to the environment. Through a process called epigenetics, the environment can influence how DNA is utilised. Instead of thinking, 'This is hereditary,' which implies that you are stuck with it, you can realise that you have the ability to change your reality, even during perimenopause.

At perimenopause, you can choose not to follow the same patterns. It can be empowering and even fun to prove everyone in the family wrong. When you choose a different path, you show that there's another way. I always ask people, 'How many in your family have had hysterectomies?' Often, the answer is, 'All my sisters, everyone.' Then I ask, 'What about you?' The response is usually, 'Oh, no, I'm the black sheep.'

It's interesting that the black sheep in the families often don't get genetic diseases. Do they have the same DNA? Yes, they do. Studies on identical twins show that 70% of what happens to them is determined by their lifestyle, thoughts, and environment. This means you have significant control over your health outcomes through your choices and mindset.

Think about it: When my book was translated into Korean, I found out that the term for menopause translates to 'no longer a woman.'

Hot Flushes, Warm Bottles

A growing number of women are currently experiencing menopause while also raising young children. The book *Hot Flushes, Warm Bottles: First Time Mothers Over Forty* by Nancy London discusses this topic. According to Dr Ellen Langer, known as the mother of mindfulness from Harvard, women who have children later in life tend to appear younger because they are frequently exposed to younger individuals. They regularly participate in events such as school plays and other activities, which helps them to stay youthful. This is called 'priming'. This constant engagement with younger generations helps maintain a youthful mindset and can even extend your lifespan.

My incredible friend, Dr. Gladys McGarey, is also featured in this book. At 103 years old, she is still teaching. She raised six kids and is now active on social media. Everyone wants to interview her, highlighting her endless passion for teaching and helping others.

She often shared stories about patients who felt tired of their daily routines, such as folding towels and making dinner, to the point where they felt like doormats. Some of these individuals became so depressed that they retreated to their beds for as long as two years before eventually recovering and moving forward with their lives.

The Importance of Self-care

During the perimenopausal stage, it can feel like every cell in your body wants to retreat into a cave for a bit—a natural urge to take some time for yourself as you reboot.

Self-care is crucial during this stage of life. Many women may not plan for it, and before they know it, they are struggling with sleep issues or noticing that their patience has worn thin. These signs are your soul's way of signalling that it's time to put your needs first. You don't need to get angry at your family members or anyone else, but you do need to recognise the importance of taking care of yourself.

If a woman drinks wine excessively, it is linked to an increased risk of breast cancer. It's important to understand that using wine or any substance to numb yourself or avoid feeling something can become a problem.

Enjoying a glass of wine with a meal occasionally is fine, but if it becomes a nightly ritual to cope, it's crucial to find other ways to soothe yourself that don't rely on external substances.

This stage is all about tuning in to your soul's needs and making self-care a priority. It's about understanding that your body is signalling for change and embracing it can lead to a more balanced and fulfilling life.

The Ascension

It's essential to understand the difference between biological age and chronological age. We are naturally designed to live much longer than we typically do, despite the challenges posed by GMOs, chemtrails, geoengineering, and other environmental factors. But here's the exciting part—we live in one of the most exciting times on Earth. Right now, we're undergoing an ascension, a transformative shift that was foretold. Surviving December 20, 2012, assured our evolution.

Throughout the history of Earth, there have been five major extinctions. This time, however, we won't be wiping ourselves out. Women experiencing perimenopause today are particularly powerful because, in a way, the entire planet is going through its own version of perimenopause. We're in a birth canal of some sort, being squeezed to tune our nervous systems in preparation for becoming a new kind of human.

Humanity is currently experiencing a major change. According to Caroline Myss, we are shifting from being focused on our physical, carbon-based form to being more attuned to energy and light. This evolution means that we are moving from our current physical form as Homo sapiens to what some call Homo luminous - a species more connected to energy, consciousness, and light.

This change reflects a shift towards higher awareness and spiritual growth, where we realise that we are not just physical beings but also beings of light and energy. This transformation marks a big step in our spiritual journey as we become more connected to the energy that supports all life.

However, not everyone will embrace this transformation. Some people will resist changing their thinking or confronting challenges head-on. They'll choose to run, hide, or play the victim. Let me tell you, the victim mindset is the easy path. It's tempting because it's supported by others—people will flock to you, and misery indeed loves company. So, if that's the path you choose, you'll find plenty of support. But understand this, you're taking the easy way out.

It's a well-worn path, but there's no growth there. You'll find a million drugs and plenty of company from people content to stay in that space. And that's okay—everyone eventually finds their way. But what you're doing and what I'm doing requires infinitely more mindfulness and strength, and the rewards are so much more satisfying, fulfilling and much more fun.

That Does Not Apply to Me

When you hear things about menopause like, 'Oh, it's the loss of sexual desire,' or whatever else they say, your mantra should be, 'That just doesn't apply to me.' That might apply to some women, but it shouldn't be your reality. Here's an example: My health insurance company used to call me every three months, offering to send someone to my home to draw blood, weigh me, and do other tests. I finally told them, 'Don't call me anymore. I'm not going to be part of your system.'

I've known for years that these so-called patient portals are just control mechanisms. They push the idea that you need your annual physical and endless tests, all based on fear. It's about catching things early, they say, but it's all fear-based, especially the fear surrounding menopause. There's so much fear attached to it, but guess what? There's a lot you can do for symptoms. I have my own product line, Amata Life, which includes Pueraria Mirifica from Thailand, and there are also bioidentical hormones for those who need them.

The most important things are your diet, exercise, and thoughts. These are the true pillars of health and well-being, not the fear-driven medical tests that so many are pushed into.

When you have too much body fat, it makes extra oestrogen and testosterone. Being stressed releases cortisol and epinephrine. The extra oestrogen in your body can be converted into additional stress hormones. If you are not physically fit, your body will transform these hormones into even more stress hormones. This creates a cycle that makes it difficult to escape from stress. Therefore, it is important to manage stress and stay fit in order to prevent this cycle and support your overall well-being.

No Magic Pill

Let's talk about this drug that's making waves—Ozempic. It's become the number one drug in the United States, costing a staggering $20,000 a year, and once you start, you're on it for life. This drug, which paralysis your stomach, is a symptom of a much bigger issue. Over 50% of people in the U.S. are overweight or obese, and while it's easy to blame big food and agriculture, we still have choices. We can still take control of our health.

I honestly believe that as we evolve, we'll move towards a healthier existence, but it's crucial to recognise that no magic pill or quick fix will solve everything. Before Ozempic, the go-to solution was bypass surgery, and how many people do I know who had that only to gain the weight back?

The transition through perimenopause involves healing past experiences so that your mind and body can experience a different awareness. The changes you make should be long-lasting because your consciousness has shifted. This is why we are here on Earth – it's a challenging place, but it's where we can make significant spiritual progress. Embrace this challenge. Your astrological chart might reveal your specific challenges, which usually involve self-healing and self-empowerment.

Finding Your Soul Family

Humanity is currently undergoing a significant change, similar to a collective version of perimenopause.

Let's talk about fear. People around the world have been traumatised by the mainstream media. As someone who has worked in the mainstream media, I understand how it operates and have learnt to ignore the fearmongering. Unfortunately, many believe everything they see and hear, thinking it's all real.

We are dividing into two groups: one that adheres to traditional beliefs and trusts everything they hear from the mainstream media and another that is becoming more conscious. Since March 2020, many people have found their soul groups. They have connected with individuals who share similar thoughts and beliefs, their star family or soul family.

An interesting phrase in the Bible from the Book of Mark goes, 'Blood is thicker than water.' I always thought that meant your blood relatives are going to be more important, but it doesn't mean that. It actually means that the blood of the covenant of the soul family is thicker than the water of the womb. Isn't that fascinating? So yes, we have our brothers and sisters, and our cultural bond is very strong—but there are aspects of our lives now that are completely different from how we grew up.

The Importance of Community

Community is more important now than it has ever been. Before 2020, I was part of a wonderful community where we danced Argentine tango. Tango is all about close connection— one heart, four legs moving in sync. But then the pandemic hit, and suddenly, everyone was terrified and wearing masks. I couldn't help but think, 'How does a mask fit into a dance that's all about close embrace?' That community just dissolved.

But out of that, something new was born. I connected with people who understood the need to question the world around us and knew the importance of coming together, even when we were told to stay apart. We embraced the idea that 'when two or more are gathered, there will I be also.' And because of what happened in March 2020, I now have more friends across the country and the world than I ever did before.

It wasn't easy. I had to step out of my comfort zone, and many people I once considered close friends drifted away. In their place, new people of all ages came into my life, and it's been incredibly exhilarating, but it required some effort.

Going Outside Your Comfort Zone

I had to step out of my comfort zone to do things I never imagined, such as boarding a plane and travelling to Tulsa, Oklahoma. Prior to this, I had never ventured into the heartland of the United States.

While in Tulsa, I met Christians for the first time. Despite being raised in the Episcopal Church, having experience playing the organ, and being confirmed, I had never been around Christians who regularly read the Bible and sincerely prayed for others. It was a completely new and truly beautiful experience for me. I didn't have any negative feelings to overcome and found it to be quite refreshing.

At the same time, I was astonished to watch how easily the people who had been in my group for years dismissed everything I'd done. For example, I was lecturing in Kansas City, and one of my friends overheard a woman in the audience say, 'Her work saved my life, but now she's gone crazy.' It was interesting to me—this person had trusted me enough to follow my advice, which had a life-saving impact on her life, but now she found it easier to dismiss everything I was saying.

On the other hand, I had another friend who heard the same things but said, 'I wanted to see where your mind went,' and we became closer than ever. This whole experience has taught me a lot about letting go.

It's about living a life guided by the dictates of your soul, not by what society expects of you. You stop making excuses for everything. There's always a temptation to stay in your own little world, right? But for me, I've become a more active Christian while still recognising the value of astrology and following people who are beautiful channels.

Some people might find the following statement controversial: Christians might say that I can't do that, and people in the channelling world might say the same. However, after menopause, you become much more interested in what you think and feel. You become more willing to admit, I could be wrong about this, and you don't need to be right or make someone else wrong. It's about accepting that everyone has their own truth in the moment. What I'm seeking now are genuine relationships, whether in the medical world or elsewhere.

Moving Forward with Forgiveness

There are still many skilled surgeons and doctors in the medical world. However, let's face it, the medical system has let humanity down in recent years. I can give you many examples to support this view. That's why we established StandFirmNow.org, a group where we collected all the evidence to support these claims.

After menopause, you undergo a shift that makes you more aware of justice and divine law. You become better at recognising what is right for you and are more willing to walk away from situations that don't align with your sense of justice.

One of my family members developed lung cancer, seemingly caused by the emotional stress of his first wife's death. Following her passing, there were conflicts over her will that caused a rift in the family. Resolving these issues required a lot of forgiveness and emotional healing. Ultimately, the family prioritised forgiveness and moving forward instead of holding on to grudges or material possessions. They chose to prevent the burden of family conflict from affecting the next generation.

Sometimes, you have to say to yourself, 'That's not right or just, but I'm not going to let it keep me from being happy or moving forward.' No matter what injustices occurred in the past, you have to find a way to let go.

Happiness Is An Inside Job

I recently spent time with a friend who lost $1.9 million in an illegal real estate deal. He did everything he could, and more, but corrupt government officials, bank officials, and lawyers were involved. Corruption seems to be everywhere. However, this is part of the planet's ascension process, like a planetary perimenopause. Consciousness is shifting, and so are we.

This realisation is why I wrote *Dodging Energy Vampires*. Throughout my career, I've realised that some people consistently drained my energy. I had to look within and ask, 'What is the part of me that feels so good to be needed by someone who is a bottomless pit?' This is a hard lesson for women. We often have these beliefs that only people who were hurt in childhood hurt others, and therefore, we need to over give to them to make them feel better. But wait a minute, there are people who are just bad seeds, and even if it's true that they were hurt in childhood, it's not my job to make them okay.

Have you ever seen those pictures from funerals, the laminated cards? I remember one from when I was a little girl, with Jesus knocking on a door that had no knob. The idea is that the door can only be opened from the inside. It's such a powerful metaphor—our happiness is an inside job. During perimenopause, this truth becomes clear. We can't rely on external things to fill us up because, eventually, the knocking from the inside starts again. External fixes are always temporary.

Guidance for Women Going Through Menopause

If I could give some guidance to a woman going through this journey right now, what would it be?

1: Maintain Normal Blood Sugar Levels

First and foremost, make sure your blood sugar levels are normal. Do whatever it takes to keep them in check because blood sugar and insulin levels cause all inflammation. Many women struggle with conditions like polycystic ovary syndrome or prediabetes, but the good news is these are completely curable. If you don't address them, they can lead to other health issues, so staying on top of your blood sugar is crucial.

2: Prioritise Self-Care and Emotional Well-Being

Spend time getting in touch with your soul. Ask yourself, 'What do I truly want?' We're often so focused on what we don't want, but it's important to think about what would feel almost too good to be true if it happened—because you deserve that and more. Every day, pay attention to your desires and what you'd like to manifest in your life. Remember, we do create our own reality on some level, so don't limit how miracles can happen. There are endless possibilities.

3: Cultivate a Positive Mindset and Community Support

Learn to recognise when someone gives you a doom-and-gloom scenario. For instance, when I was 42 and writing *Women's Bodies, Women's Wisdom*, my literary agent told me, 'You're not getting any younger, you know.'

That same agent is long gone, and since then, I've written three New York Times bestsellers. When people say these things to you, laugh it off. Don't let their negativity get to you.

4. Stop Saying Your Age

If someone asks you how old you are, You could say something like, 'My wisdom age is 350, but my biological age is 35.' Or if you're at the gym, just put in an age that feels right for you—like 40—because those machines often calculate in a way that assumes a decline as you age. I've been doing this for decades. And if someone asks your age directly, like a man did once to me while I was biking in Santa Barbara, respond with, 'What's your real question?' It shifts the conversation and keeps the focus on what truly matters.

What Gives Me Joy?

Here's what brings me joy: Beautiful music—especially romantic film scores that touch the soul, like this one: Hanz Zimmer- Chevaliers De Sangreal Live in Prague. I also find such peace and connection in praise music, which I often start my day with, grounding myself in gratitude and grace. Here's one of my favourites: Gratitude – Brandam Lake/Moment.

Another source of daily delight is what I lovingly refer to as 'God's Internet,' also known as the Law of Attraction. Those thousand little synchronicities each day remind us of the divine order of things—stories of people healing, finding love, and, yes, even the joy of watching funny animal videos! These small, magical moments always bring a smile to my face.

And let's not forget the joy of laughter! Any chance to laugh is a gift. These are the things that light up my life.

Where to Learn More About Dr. Christiane Northrup's Work

To explore Dr. Christiane Northrup's extensive work on women's health and wellness, visit her official website at drnorthrup.com. There, you'll find a wealth of resources, articles, and insights on topics ranging from menopause to holistic health.

Dr. Northrup shares regular updates and articles through her Substack platforms, where she dives deeper into current health topics and her unique perspectives on wellness.

You can follow her on True North Doctor Substack at www.truenorthdr.substack.com for her latest insights. Additionally, she connects with her community on her Telegram channel, offering a space for open discussions and support. You can join her Telegram channel at t.me/DrChristianeNorthrup.

For those interested in health products by Dr. Northrup, visit www.amatalife.com. She offers a line of supplements specifically designed to support women's hormonal health and vitality. Learn more about these products on her website.

These platforms provide various ways to engage with Dr. Northrup's teachings, from her foundational books to her latest insights, all aimed at empowering women on their journey to optimal health and wellbeing.

My Reflections After
Our Conversation

I was left speechless. I had just met the woman who had influenced my growth journey—Dr. Northrup. She guided me through some of my life's heaviest and most challenging times. Her laughter lifted my spirits when I was down, and when I felt weak, she gave me the strength to believe in myself. Dr Northrup encouraged me to choose a different path, one less travelled, and in doing so, I found a renewed sense of freedom, even during the nearly two years I spent in lockdown in Melbourne, Australia—the most locked-down city in the world during the pandemic.

When I was approaching my mid-40s in 2015, I started feeling the impact of aging in a society that values youth. This growing awareness led me to Dr. Northrup's book, Goddesses Never Age. As I approached my 48th birthday, her insights completely transformed my perspective on aging. I realised that I no longer wanted to waste energy chasing after youth, a game I had played before. Instead, I decided to focus on my health, eat well, take care of myself, and let whatever comes from that be enough. Dr. Northrup's wisdom helped me navigate this phase of life without getting trapped in the 'cage of aging.' as she says in her book.

My research into the beauty industry only reinforced this decision. It's a multibillion-dollar machine that thrives on our insecurities, keeping us on a never-ending treadmill of external validation. The numbers we get caught up in—our age, weight, and bank balance—can easily become another cage. There have been moments when I get enslaved in that mindset, but I've learnt to stay grounded by prioritising my overall well-being.

Every day, I tune into my body to determine its needs. This could mean walking, practising yoga, doing Pilates, weight training, or simply taking a day of rest. I've come to understand that true contentment comes from within rather than from external factors such as wealth, weight or appearance. By maintaining a balanced approach to both diet and exercise, I feel much better. Overall, my mind is sharper, my mood is improved, and I'm more present for my family. When I make less healthy choices, I quickly feel the consequences, such as hot flushes, bloating, and poor digestion. However, I've learnt to get back on track swiftly. Recognising the importance of consistency, especially as a post-menopausal woman, has helped me make choices that support my long-term health.

Embracing Dr. Northrup's teachings and focusing on my well-being have allowed me to live a more fulfilling life. I'm no longer chasing after youth or external validation; I'm cultivating happiness from within. This shift in perspective has made all the difference.

Dr. Northrup talked about Ozempic, the leading weight loss drug in the USA, which encouraged me to look into the size of the weight loss industry. The weight loss industry is very large and relies on our focus on achieving the ideal weight. It is valued at over $250 billion and continues to grow every year. In the United States alone, more than $70 billion is spent annually on weight loss products and services. China's market exceeds $40 billion, Japan's is around $20 billion, Germany's is about $15 billion, and Brazil contributes another $10 billion. Even countries like the United Kingdom, France, and Australia are significant players, with markets valued at $8 billion, $7 billion, and $5 billion, respectively.

But here's the thing: this entire system feeds on our insecurities, keeping us locked in a cycle of chasing quick fixes rather than finding real, lasting solutions. If you follow the money, it becomes clear how much this industry profits from making us feel like we're never quite good enough.

The beauty and anti-aging industries follow similar patterns. These industries are massive, with the global beauty industry valued at over $500 billion and the anti-aging market expected to reach nearly $300 billion by 2026. The top 10 countries leading in beauty spending are:

- United States - The largest market, estimated at over $90 billion annually.

- China - Rapidly growing, with a market size exceeding $60 billion.

- Japan - A major player in the beauty market, worth around $35 billion.

- Brazil - Leading in Latin America, with a market size of approximately $30 billion.

- Germany - Europe's largest beauty market, valued at about $20 billion.

- South Korea - Known for its innovative products, with a market size of over $15 billion.

- India - An emerging market with significant growth, valued at around $14 billion.

- France - The home of luxury beauty, with a market size of roughly $13 billion.

- United Kingdom - A strong European market worth around $12 billion.

- Italy - Another key European market with a value close to $10 billion.

Yet, despite all these products and the billions spent, are we any happier? The data suggests otherwise. What does that tell us? These industries are designed to keep us in these cages—constantly striving, never truly satisfied.

Breaking free from these cycles isn't just about making different choices; it's about embracing a whole new perspective on yourself. It takes courage to look inward, connect deeply with your true self, and realise that you are already enough, just as you are. What if we could let go of the constant need for more? Imagine stepping back from the chaos and embracing that your worth isn't tied to a number or societal standard.

This journey requires questioning societal norms and embracing authentic living. Are you ready to explore a different path? Are you ready to break free from the limitations imposed by aging, much like freeing yourself from the matrix? The challenge is real, but so are the rewards.

And here's the magic: When you embrace this mindset, something truly enchanting unfolds. You begin to see the world through a different lens, realising that you don't need to chase perfection because you're already whole. Life becomes richer, not dictated by numbers or societal pressures, but by your own inner truth. This freedom brings a sense of peace and joy, reconnecting you with your deeper self, where true transformation occurs. That's where the real magic lies— in the freedom to be unapologetically you. That's the wonder of menopause.

Reflecting on my conversation with Dr. Christiane Northrup, I was struck by her contagious laughter, light, and wisdom. She seemed to carry an understanding far beyond her years, as if she had been on this planet before and grasped what was truly important. Learning from her has been a privilege and has given me the courage to continue on my path, knowing that I'm not alone in this life journey. We all need someone to guide us at times, and her presence has inspired strength and freedom on my journey.

Reflection Activity:
During Menopause

Staying active during menopause is essential for maintaining your health and well-being. Here are some practical tips and activities from Dr. Northrup to help you navigate this transformative period with ease and vitality.

Daily Practices for a Balanced and Empowered Life

Life's journey is filled with opportunities for growth, reflection, and connection. We can create a more balanced and fulfilling life by focusing on key areas such as health, self-awareness, and community. The following activities are designed to help you nurture your body, mind, and spirit. Take each step with intention, knowing that small changes can lead to transformations.

Activity 1: Maintain Normal Blood Sugar

- **Get Tested:** Regularly check your sugar and insulin levels.

- **Prompt:** Schedule a blood sugar test with your doctor this month.

- **Diet and Exercise:** Control your levels through a balanced diet and regular exercise to reduce inflammation.

- **Prompt:** Plan three healthy weekly meals and choose an exercise activity each day.

Activity 2: Connect with Your Soul:

- **Daily Reflection:** Spend a few minutes each day thinking about what you truly want. Reflecting daily helps align your actions with your true desires.

- **Prompt:** Write down one thing you desire in your journal every morning.

- **Visualisation:** Imagine yourself achieving your desires and knowing you deserve them. Visualisation reinforces the belief that your goals are attainable.

- **Prompt:** Spend five minutes each evening visualising your goals as if they have already been achieved.

Activity 3: Dismiss Negative Scenarios:

- **Stay Positive:** Remember that negative predictions don't have to apply to you. Reframing thoughts can reduce stress and promote mental well-being.

- **Prompt:** Identify one negative thought you've had recently and reframe it positively.

- **Adopt a Mantra:** Use affirmations like, 'That just doesn't apply to me,' to counter negativity.

- **Prompt:** Repeat your chosen mantra three times each day.

Activity 3: Embrace Your Wisdom Age:

- **Change Your Mindset:** Focus on your wisdom age rather than your chronological age. Your experiences contribute to your wisdom and inner growth.

- **Prompt:** Reflect on your experiences and note how they contribute to your wisdom.

- **Confident Responses:** When asked your age, consider saying, 'My wisdom age reflects my experiences; my biological age is just a number.'

- **Prompt:** Practice this response in front of a mirror.

Activity 4: Listen to Your Body

- **Rest and Recovery:** Ensure you get enough rest and recovery time. Rest is essential for maintaining overall health and well-being.

- **Prompt:** Plan a relaxing activity for each evening this week.

Activity 5: Community Connection:

- **Build New Connections:** Form new communities and support networks to stay motivated and engaged. Consider what you need in a community—support, shared interests, growth—and seek groups that align with these needs.

- **Prompt:** Join a local group, women's circle, or online community that interests you.

Concluding Thoughts

As you incorporate these practices into your daily life, remember that true transformation happens gradually. Be patient with yourself and celebrate each small victory along the way. By taking these intentional steps, you're nurturing a life of balance, fulfilment, and empowerment. Trust the journey and enjoy the process of becoming your most authentic self.

CHAPTER 6

Dr Vandana Shiva

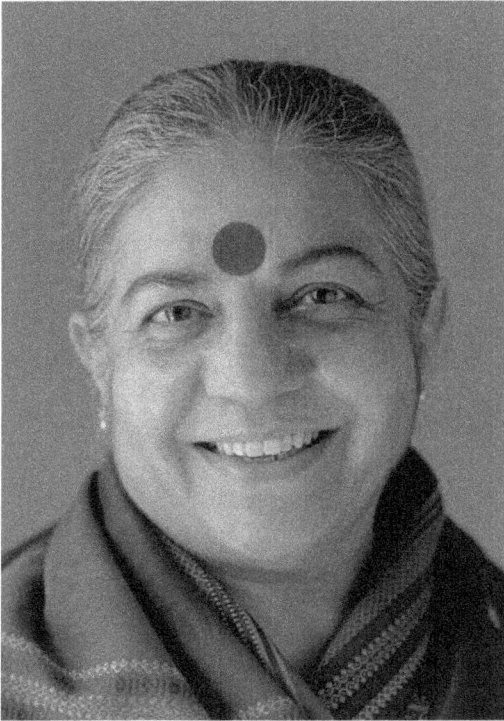

The Warrior

Discovering Dr. Vandana Shiva

I first encountered Dr. Vandana Shiva's work while searching for a deeper understanding of the connection between our natural environment and human life cycles. I had always been passionate about sustainable living and mindful consumption, but something about her philosophy on seeds, agriculture, and the Earth struck a chord. Dr Shiva's insights weren't just about the food we eat or the environmental consequences of industrial farming, she spoke about the cycles that sustain all life and the inherent wisdom of nature.

I discovered her through her book *Stolen Harvest*, a powerful exploration of how corporate control over agriculture disrupts the delicate balance of life. The way she illustrated that small-scale farmers—especially women—hold the key to a sustainable future resonated deeply with me. Her words awakened something inside me. I had never considered the significance of seeds so deeply before: how they embody the potential for life, regeneration, and continuity. This simple concept began to reshape not only how I viewed food and agriculture but also how I understood the different phases of my own life.

Dr. Shiva's teachings struck me on an intensely personal level, especially as I reflected on the natural cycles of womanhood, including the transition of menopause. Her philosophy helped me see that just as a seed holds the promise of new life and renewal, menopause is not a closing chapter but a stage of transformation—one of wisdom, reflection, and the potential for new growth. I began to view this phase of life as a time for planting new seeds of experience, knowledge, and insight that would take root and flourish in the next stage of my journey.

One particular afternoon, I stood in my garden, holding seeds in my hand, and the realisation washed over me: menopause, like these seeds, was not an ending but a new beginning. Just as seeds lie dormant before they sprout in fertile soil, I, too, was entering a phase filled with possibilities. This realisation was not just intellectual but emotional, spiritual, and deeply personal.

Dr Shiva's work reminded me of the growing organic farming movements, where small-scale farmers fight to preserve traditional farming methods and seed diversity. Like the farmers in India whom Dr Shiva defends, these local heroes resist the industrialisation of agriculture, keeping our agricultural heritage and ecosystems alive. Her teachings revealed that the seed is far more than a metaphor—it's a powerful symbol of resilience, renewal, and the ability to thrive in the face of adversity.

Dr. Vandana Shiva's work opened my eyes to the interconnectedness of all things: the Earth, the food we eat, and the life cycles we experience as women. Her message has shaped how I approach my relationship with nature and honour life's different phases.

Introduction to Dr. Vandana Shiva

Dr. Vandana Shiva is a globally renowned environmental activist, ecofeminist, and tireless advocate for sustainable agriculture. With a PhD in physics, specialising in quantum theory, her path took a transformative turn when she left academia to dedicate herself to defending biodiversity and advocating the rights of small-scale farmers. Dr. Shiva's work highlights the sacred relationship between humans and nature, emphasising the critical importance of seed sovereignty and the dangers posed by corporate control over agriculture.

In 1982, she founded the Research Foundation for Science, Technology, and Ecology, and in 1991, she launched Navdanya, a movement committed to protecting biodiversity, preserving indigenous farming practices, and promoting organic agriculture. Through Navdanya, Dr. Shiva has fought relentlessly against the spread of genetically modified organisms (GMOs) and industrial agriculture, which she argues disrupts the delicate balance of nature and threatens the livelihoods of farmers worldwide.

Her activism is rooted in her belief that seeds are not merely commodities but the very essence of life. Dr. Shiva has written extensively on the interconnectedness of women, nature, and the cycles of life in works such as Staying Alive, Monocultures of the Mind, and Soil Not Oil. Her philosophy challenges the exploitation of both women and nature, asserting that true sustainability comes from respecting and nurturing the Earth's natural systems.

Dr Shiva's efforts have earned her numerous accolades, including the Right Livelihood Award, the Sydney Peace Prize, and the MIDORI Prize for Biodiversity. Her advocacy inspires individuals worldwide to reconnect with nature, respect biodiversity, and honour the cycles of life that sustain both the Earth and humanity.

As we move into the following conversation, Dr Shiva's work serves as a framework for exploring the connections between nature's cycles and the human experience, particularly the journey of womanhood and the transformative power of menopause.

"We are either going to have a future where women lead the way to make peace with the Earth

or we are not going to have a human future at all."

Dr Vandana Shiva

A Conversation with
Dr Vandana Shiva

The Forests of the Himalayas
and the Path to Physics

I grew up surrounded by the forests of the Himalayas—nature was all I knew. My school didn't emphasise physics much, but that changed when I picked up a book by Einstein. His ideas captivated me, and I felt a calling to pursue physics. I remember being in Canada, preparing for discussions on quantum theory and my thesis, feeling like I was at a crossroads. I could have easily stayed on the safe, predictable path of quantum theory, which I loved.

But I couldn't ignore the other puzzles around me—questions about how science, technology, and society are interconnected. I thought I'd spend a few years understanding these connections, and decades later, I'm still trying to figure it out.

From Physics to Activism—The Turning Point

People ask me all the time how I went from studying quantum physics to becoming an environmental activist. But for me, it didn't feel like a big leap. In quantum theory, everything is interconnected, and that's something I've carried with me into my work. So, in a way, I never really left quantum physics behind—it just became a broader way of looking at the world and understanding how things are connected.

The true turning point came when I visited my favourite forest before leaving for Canada. When I arrived, it was gone. **The place I loved, the trees that had been there my whole life, had disappeared.** It felt like I had lost a piece of myself. While waiting for the bus, I had a conversation with a local chaiwala (tea seller) who told me about Chipko, a movement where women were standing up to stop deforestation. These women knew the land deeply and they were fighting to protect it.

That moment stuck with me. Even as I continued my PhD, I couldn't ignore the pull of activism. During every school break, I volunteered with the Chipko movement, and over time, it became just as important to me as my academic work. They weren't separate, they were part of the same journey.

The Bindi
A Symbol of Power and Connection

As a child, I was told the bindi on my forehead symbolised marriage, but I never thought much of it. It wasn't until I came across a book about **the Sri Chakra—the Chakra of Feminine Power**—that I started to see it differently. The bindi represents something far more powerful than I realised. In Indian philosophy, everything is connected in diverse ways, and there are so many ways to represent ideas—through icons, mantras, or geometric forms like the Sri Chakra.

What struck me is how everything in nature is connected. A line, for example, is just a moving dot, and from these simple shapes, we can create everything in the world. This idea reminded me of my studies in quantum theory, where one small particle holds the potential for endless possibilities. That's when I began to see the bindi not just as a cultural symbol but as a representation of holding the world within us.

Returning to India
A Turning Point in my life in Punjab

After finishing my PhD in 1982, I decided to return to India. A lot of people I studied with chose to stay abroad, but for me, coming back home felt like the right thing to do. I wanted to be close to my family and contribute meaningfully. At that point, I wasn't entirely sure what direction to take. Should I stick with quantum theory or look deeper into the issues we were facing as a society? Eventually, I joined the Institute of Science and later the Institute of Management, where I started studying how science and technology intersect with societal problems.

In 1982, shortly after my return, the Ministry of Environment invited me to conduct a major study on mining in the Doon Valley—my home. This project held deep personal significance, especially as I was grieving the loss of my mother and had just become a parent myself. Our study was used in a Supreme Court case, and the Court ruled in favour of shutting down the mines. Their decision was based on the principle that when commerce threatens life, commerce must cease for life to continue. This landmark ruling was grounded in Article 21 of the Indian Constitution, which guarantees the fundamental right to life.

The Violence of the Green Revolution
A Deepening Commitment to Agriculture

At that time, the United Nations University requested that I investigate the rise of global resource conflicts. I had personally witnessed the disappearance of forests, rivers, and lands. Grassroots movements were emerging in various places. The United Nations (UN) provided funding for a five-year study, a rare opportunity at the time. This allowed me to thoroughly examine every movement related to forests, rivers, and mining by directly engaging with the people involved.

Then, in 1984, Punjab erupted in violence. I studied there, doing my Masters in particle physics, and I remembered it as a peaceful and prosperous land. But in 1984, it had turned into a place of deep conflict. I told the UN that I wanted to study what was happening. That led to my book, *The Violence of the Green Revolution*. The more I learned, the clearer it became that the Green Revolution was about selling war chemicals, not about feeding people sustainably. That realisation changed everything for me.

I am committed to learning, studying, and growing for my personal development, not for anyone else or external reasons. When I realised that the Green Revolution was primarily about selling war chemicals, I knew I had to find a nonviolent approach to farming. This transition was a significant leap, but I trusted my conscience and made those changes. Since 1984, I have dedicated myself to farms and sustainable agriculture.

During a difficult time in Punjab, many farmers lost their lives in fires and violence. This deeply affected me and was a major reason I decided to create Navdanya.

The Birth of Navdanya
A Response to a Global Crisis

'Nav' means 'new' or 'nine,' and 'danya' means 'gift.' When I asked the farmer why he grew nine crops, he explained, 'Nine crops because there are nine planets. The diversity of cops in my field, like the diversity of food we need for a healthy life, is interconnected. I am taking care of this harmony.' His words encapsulated the balance and interconnectedness that Navdanya would come to represent.

A Wake-Up Call

The movement to start saving seeds gained momentum during a UN meeting on biotechnology, which took place before the introduction of GMOs in 1992. During this meeting, industry leaders—primarily from the chemical industry—made a startling statement: 'We are very poor. We need to make more money, and chemicals aren't enough. We must turn to seeds as a source of income.' They planned to use genetic engineering to patent seeds, which horrified me. I remember thinking, 'But a patent is for an invention. You don't invent a seed. A seed is the continuity of life.'

It became even more concerning when they stated, 'It's not enough to introduce these laws in the industrial world. We must use international laws, like those under GATT (General Agreement on Tariffs and Trade), which later became the World Trade Organisation (WTO), to prevent farmers from saving seeds.' This directly attacked one of humanity's highest duties: to preserve life. They were attempting to criminalise a sacred act and falsely claim they had created life itself.

The Decision to Save Seeds
A Leap of Conscience

On my return flight, I made a decision. I didn't know exactly how I would do it, but I knew I had to save seeds. I had no prior experience in agriculture, but I learned. I decided to closely follow the developments in genetic engineering, patents, and the WTO, knowing these tools would further the corporate control agenda.

Since then, I've worked with the UN to help draft biosafety laws and assisted in shaping laws in my own country. I affirm that plants, animals, and seeds are not human inventions and cannot be patented. Patents are for true inventions, not for the continuity of life.

Navdanya's Impact

Today, Navdanya stands as a testament to the power of grassroots movements. We have established over 50 community seed banks, and every farmer we encouraged to preserve seeds is now prospering. Unfortunately, many farmers who were forced into dependence on patented seeds found themselves in debt, leading to tragic suicides. We have studied these impacts and continue to fight for a nonviolent, sustainable path forward in agriculture. Through Navdanya, we are helping to restore the balance between humanity and nature—one seed, one farmer, one field at a time.

The Concept of 'God Move Over'

When I talk about GMOs and use the phrase 'God move over,' I'm pointing to what's happening in the seed industry. Today, just a few big companies control about 60% of commercial seeds worldwide, mostly because they hold patents.

Take Monsanto, for example. How did they become so dominant in the seed sector? They didn't invent something entirely new. Instead, they acquired research from other companies, used patents to secure control and, in doing so, became a powerful force in agriculture.

What does it mean to patent a seed? A seed represents the evolution of life and the innovation of countless generations of farmers. Indian farmers, for instance, have evolved 200,000 rice varieties from a single type of grass. Mexican farmers created thousands of corn varieties from a wild plant called teosinte. This incredible diversity, which we benefit from today, is the result of the combined creativity of nature and the wisdom passed down through generations of farmers and our ancestors.

When the industry claims to have patented seeds, it's essentially saying, 'We are the creators of life.' It is appropriating the natural process of creation and the contributions made by farmers over millennia. In effect, a patent on life—a patent on a seed—suggests that there is no divine creator and that the industry itself is the creator.

This is why I say that patents on seeds and the genetically modified organisms that facilitate these patents are essentially a message to the world: '**GMO: God move over.**' It's a way of saying that corporations are now in control of life itself, pushing aside the natural, divine process of creation in favour of their industrial, profit-driven agenda.

The Disappearance of Biodiversity
A Global Crisis

The main threat posed by GMOs is their impact on biodiversity. Natural processes thrive on biodiversity, encouraging a wide variety of species and plants. However, genetic engineering often leads to monoculture, where only a single type of crop is cultivated. This lack of diversity undermines ecosystems, which depend on a balance of species to remain healthy and resilient.

Although GMOs were initially promoted as a solution for growing food in harsh environments, like deserts or even on the Moon, their actual success has been much more limited.

The first generation of GMOs focused on two main traits: crops that resist the herbicide glyphosate (such as Roundup-ready plants) and plants that produce Bacillus thuringiensis (Bt) toxin, which acts as a pesticide. However, even these advancements are showing signs of failure. For instance, pests have started to develop resistance to Bt cotton, a problem Monsanto, one of the biggest GMO producers, has acknowledged.

GMOs not only threaten biodiversity but also severely degrade soil health. Studies on Bt crops have shown that they fail to attract pollinators, which are crucial for ecosystems. Within the first four years of planting Bt crops, 60% of the beneficial microorganisms in the soil are destroyed, turning fertile land into barren deserts. This degradation undermines the Earth's natural fertility, pushing farmers to rely even more on chemical inputs and compromising the long-term sustainability of agriculture.

Beyond environmental destruction, GMOs have created an economic stranglehold on farmers. The driving force behind GMOs is not feeding the world but generating profits. Traditional seeds that once cost farmers 5 to 10 rupees now sell for as much as 4,000 rupees due to corporate control. This immense cost has pushed many farmers into debt. Tragically, in countries like India, this debt has led to a spike in farmer suicides, with many unable to escape the financial burden imposed by GMO seed pricing.

Another pressing issue concerns the health risks of GMOs. The chemical industry, now intertwined with the seed industry, has attempted to downplay the dangers, claiming that the toxins in Bt crops degrade quickly. However, studies show that Bt toxin has been found in the bloodstreams of pregnant women and their foetuses. This raises significant concerns about the long-term health implications of consuming genetically modified food, especially when these toxins accumulate within the human body over time.

The Lasting Impact of Colonialism on Women and the Earth

Colonialism, whether in Africa, India, or 85% of the world colonised by the British, played a significant role in disrupting natural relationships. While the Spanish often used religion to assert control, the British relied on violence and manipulation of knowledge. They redefined the Earth as lifeless and depicted women as passive beings.

This shift is closely linked to Francis Bacon, often called the father of modern science. Bacon's work, *The Birth of Masculine Time*, marked the dawn of modern science and introduced the notion that the precolonial world was 'effeminate and weak.' This new 'masculine time' sought to dominate the Earth, viewing it solely as a resource, while women with knowledge of plants and healing were persecuted as witches. Indigenous knowledge—ranging from steelmaking to smallpox vaccinations—was appropriated and subsequently banned in their lands. For instance, smallpox vaccination, originally an Indian practice, was adopted by the British, presented to the Royal Society, and then prohibited in India.

The Connection Between Earth, Seeds, Soil, and Women

Colonial violence fractured the natural connection between the Earth, seeds, soil, and women. Despite centuries of suppression, this bond has endured. Like the Earth, women are inherently creative forces—they give life, nurture growth, and sustain communities. This creativity is deeply tied to the Earth, a constant source of life and abundance.

When I speak of symbols like the bindi or paintings, I refer to the inherent creativity in everything. Just as the Earth continuously regenerates, women possess a life-giving power that mirrors this regenerative energy. Colonialism sought to sever this connection, but it persisted through women's care for their families, communities, and the Earth.

Reviving Women's Role as Caregivers of the Earth

Throughout history, women have been the primary caregivers of life—both for their families and the Earth. Despite centuries of oppression, they have preserved the knowledge and creativity necessary to sustain life. Whether through preserving seeds, growing food, or nurturing future generations, women's role in caring for the Earth remains essential.

This enduring connection between women and the Earth reflects a deep historical tradition. Women have always been at the heart of life-giving processes. To relearn how to care for the planet, we must look to these women and their knowledge, which has been preserved and passed down through generations. They hold a vision of humanity that is rooted in care, love, and community, offering an alternative to the violence, domination, and greed perpetuated by colonialism.

Learning from Ancient Matriarchal Societies, Women and the Earth

Historically, all societies cared for the Earth, but colonialism fundamentally disrupted this relationship. Colonialism laid the groundwork for capitalist patriarchy, displacing men to work in plantations and mines while dispossessing Indigenous people of their lands. In this upheaval, women were often left behind to care for the Earth and the children. Although forced upon them, this responsibility allowed women to retain what truly matters—sustaining life and nurturing the Earth.

A Manifesto for Change
Making Peace with the Earth

Years ago, I founded the Diverse Women for Diversity movement to resist harmful global practices, such as those promoted by the WTO, and to protect biodiversity. Through this movement, we produced the manifesto Making Peace with the Earth, which outlines the principles women have safeguarded and lived by for generations. These principles reflect an understanding of life—both ethically and scientifically.

The manifesto seeks to restore balance by advocating for a worldview that respects the Earth as a living system and recognises women's essential role as caretakers. By reviving these values, we can address the global environmental crises and heal the planet and ourselves.

Uniting Women Globally
Addressing the Food Supply Crisis

Women must unite globally to tackle the growing crisis of compromised food supplies and sustainability. Their natural understanding of diversity—whether in the seeds they preserve, the food systems they nurture, or the knowledge they safeguard—is vital. By weaving this diversity into daily life, women can transform the food systems currently depleting the Earth and human health.

The principles outlined in Making Peace with the Earth are central to this effort. They offer a framework for collective action, bringing women together globally to address the critical challenges we face. Through cooperation and shared wisdom, women can lead the way in creating sustainable, resilient food systems.

Practising Sustainability in Daily Life

While global unity is essential, individual actions also play a crucial role. Women can contribute to a more sustainable and just food system by cultivating diverse seeds, preparing sustainable food, and sharing knowledge within their communities. These small, daily actions allow women to continue honouring the Earth and ensuring the wellbeing of future generations.

By practising sustainability in their everyday lives, women embody the life-giving, regenerative energy that has long been tied to their connection with the Earth. In doing so, they preserve their ancient role as caregivers and create a hopeful future for all of humanity.

The Great Reset
A Crisis Turned into Control

The idea of the Great Reset needs careful examination. This concept gained widespread attention when a book with the same title was released at the peak of the global pandemic when people were locked down and dealing with unprecedented crises. Labelling that moment as an 'opportunity' shows the deeper issue.

When you create a crisis and then use it to impose a new system of control, you're taking advantage of people's vulnerabilities. Millions lost their livelihoods, entire economies collapsed, and even now, people haven't fully recovered from the aftermath of the pandemic. The very word Reset' implies that those in power think they have already 'set the stage' and now wish to reset it as they see fit, controlling society's direction. That's where the problem begins.

Colonialism, Control, and Exploitation

This kind of thinking reflects a colonial mindset— where free societies, free individuals, and even natural organisms are supposed to evolve independently but are controlled and dictated by an external power. Historically, this kind of interference has caused societies to break down. We've seen this through the so-called 'development' pushed by institutions like the World Bank and the International Monetary Fund (IMF). These organisations have twisted the world in harmful ways.

For example, take what happened around Bangalore, where farmers were pushed to grow eucalyptus, a crop completely unsuitable for semiarid lands. This resulted from World Bank policies, which ultimately destroyed local environments.

Global Institutions and Their Destructive Role

Whenever we examine major environmental or economic crises in the Global South (the UN Trade and Development define the Global South comprises Africa, Latin America and the Caribbean, Asia (excluding Israel, Japan, and South Korea), and Oceania (excluding Australia and New Zealand), the same players always appear—the World Bank, the IMF, and, more recently, the WTO. These organisations, along with the World Economic Forum (WEF), are promoting a form of globalisation that serves only the interests of the powerful.

The result has been the rise of a global elite—the infamous 1%—who control most of the world's wealth, leaving 99% of people struggling. Corporations like BlackRock and Vanguard control vast shares of global industries, land, and housing markets. When Bayer bought Monsanto, it wasn't just a simple business transaction. Through research, I discovered that BlackRock and Vanguard control Bayer and Monsanto. This shows how the rich continue accumulating power, using these companies to take control of our food systems and lives.

When these powerful organisations talk about the Great Reset, they're discussing the colonisation of what little control ordinary people have left. It's about reshaping the world to benefit the elite while taking away our freedom. The Great Reset is far more than an economic plan—it's about controlling resources, technology, and even our everyday lives.

However, the Great Reset can also serve as a wake-up call—a signal that humanity must reclaim its freedom. We can resist these control systems and rebuild a world where the Earth, communities, and individuals are respected and valued. This is a moment for us to seek freedom again and to create a future based on justice, balance, and respect for all life.

Vision for Sustainable Agriculture and Environmental Activism

I envision a world where diversity thrives—small farmers are at the heart of our food systems. In my experience, small farmers produce more food, do less harm to the environment, and create culture in a way that large industrial farms simply cannot. Instead of relying on globalised trade in junk and poison-laden foods, I see a future where local food economies flourish, where biodiversity is celebrated and sustains us. By nurturing biodiversity, we can cultivate diverse food systems that nourish both the planet and its people, respecting the inherent abundance of nature.

In this world, hunger and malnutrition will no longer exist because there is no scarcity when we work with nature. The solution to climate change begins with this same principle—biodiversity. The more diversity we nurture, the less harm we do to the climate. It's all interconnected. Biodiversity is the foundation for health as well. Doctors now acknowledge that the gut microbiome is central to our health, and the diversity of our food is essential to maintaining it. Everything is linked: the soil, the food we eat, our health, and the planet's health.

Industrial agriculture can never replicate the love and care small farmers invest in their food. Mass-produced food cannot carry the love and attention that goes into every seed and crop planted by farmers. Big companies can't replicate this, no matter how efficient or high-tech their systems are. This love makes all the difference, it's what nourishes the body and soul.

The Push for 'Farming Without Farmers' and Its Consequences

A couple of years ago, Bill Gates and his network began promoting slogans like 'Farming without farmers' and

'Food without farms.' This rhetoric reflects an alarming agenda for pushing small farmers out and replacing real, naturally grown food with lab-engineered alternatives. Gates' agenda is advancing rapidly, underpinned by claims that synthetic food solves climate change. However, this narrative is both unscientific and misleading.

First, replacing natural farming with lab-grown food would worsen climate issues, not improve them. Studies show synthetic food production could generate up to 25 times more emissions than traditional farming. Emissions are the root cause of climate change, and substituting real farms with food labs would only intensify the problem.

Secondly, ultra-processed food, which would come from such labs, is directly linked to the rise of diet-related diseases. The mass production of these foods already contributes to widespread health issues and turning all food into 'lab food' would exacerbate this. This shift isn't a solution to climate or health challenges, it is a disaster for human health and the environment.

Moreover, this agenda represents a direct threat to small farmers, who have nurtured the land and grown food with care for generations. We must respect these farmers and the real food they produce. As a mother lovingly prepares meals for her family, farmers grow vegetables and crops with that same love and dedication for their communities. Replacing this deep connection with lab-produced food strips away the care and humanity that sustains our bodies and our environment.

For the future of food and the planet, we must support and stand in solidarity with real farmers. They are the guardians of biodiversity, food security, and cultural heritage. Through our collective efforts, we can ensure that small farmers continue to thrive and that real food—grown with love and respect—has a future.

Reflecting on the Four Industrial Revolutions

Technological advancements have transformed how we live, work, and interact with the world. These shifts, known as industrial revolutions, have marked major societal turning points. As we navigate the Fourth Industrial Revolution, it's important to understand how these previous revolutions shaped our world today.

The first industrial revolution was driven by coal and fertilisers, which laid the foundation for mechanising agriculture and industry. The second industrial revolution introduced advancements in genetic engineering, changing how we interacted with nature and altering the course of human development. The third revolution brought these innovations together by merging genetic engineering with advanced tools and digital technology, paving the way for automation and global connectivity.

Now, in the Fourth Industrial Revolution, we are seeing the convergence of all the previous ones. This era still relies on fertilisers, fossil fuels, and biotechnology, but what sets it apart is the way technology is being integrated into every aspect of life. Financial technologies (FinTech), for example, are being used to push for digital IDs, digital currencies, and widespread software systems. This merger of biotechnology, information technology, financial technologies, and fossil fuel industries is creating a massive surveillance system—one that could potentially be used to control and, in some ways, enslave us.

Living a Sovereign Life in a Programmed World

In a world dominated by fear and scarcity, returning to a culture of abundance is the solution. Food is our most fundamental connection to the Earth; its quality can nourish or harm us. If we begin to care for the planet and nourish our bodies with clean, healthy food, we start dismantling the systems that seek to control us through food dependency.

This journey towards abundance begins with small, personal actions—choosing organic, saving seeds, and supporting real farmers who grow food with love and care. These choices nurture our health and ensure that the planet remains healthy and abundant for future generations.

I encourage everyone to take these steps and delve deeper into sustainable farming and seed-saving principles. At Navdanya, we offer various courses, and our farm is always open for those who wish to see these principles in action. It's about making personal choices that collectively have a global impact, preserving life in its most natural and abundant form.

Embracing the Freedom of Menopause
A Personal Reflection

If I were to offer any advice to women navigating menopause, it would be this: trust yourself. Every woman understands her own body and journey better than anyone else. While I'm not one to tell others what to do, I can share what menopause meant to me and how it felt in my life.

For me, **menopause was a celebration of freedom**. It wasn't just a physical change but a release from the small, practical concerns I no longer had to consider. For example, I no longer needed to stock up on sanitary products before heading into the field, far from any store. It was a sense of liberation.

Spiritually, menopause didn't feel like a significant shift for me because I had always lived with a deep connection to both the Earth and my community. I had long been rooted in my work for the planet, and menopause didn't take me in a new direction. Rather, it felt like a continuation—a deepening of the path I had been walking all along. Menopause seemed to invite me to step more fully into my purpose, with the wisdom I had accumulated over the years becoming even more central to my work.

For me, menopause wasn't a dramatic transformation but a natural evolution. It brought a new sense of freedom, allowing me to continue my life's work with greater purpose and clarity. It wasn't about change but rather about embracing the journey I had been on with a renewed sense of empowerment and liberation.

What Brings Me Joy

When asked what gives me joy, the answer is simple: life itself. I think back to when my child was born and the experience of another life coming into the world through my body. That deep sense of interconnectedness and respect for each individual as a unique being has always been a source of wonder for me.

My joy now comes from nurturing living systems—the seeds, plants, and communities I work with every day. Caring for these life forms and helping them thrive brings satisfaction. The simplest acts of nurturing life are the most rewarding.

Final Thoughts and Invitation to Navdanya

As we close this discussion, I want to extend a heartfelt invitation. If you're eager to learn more about food sovereignty, ecofeminism, or the importance of saving seeds, I encourage you to visit our website at Navdanya.org. We offer a variety of courses, including one I teach each March on ecofeminism. You're also welcome to visit our farm, stay with us, and participate in internships or hands-on courses to experience this way of living firsthand.

It would be an honour to meet you, share this wisdom, and work together towards a more conscious, connected way of living. Thank you for being a part of this important conversation, and I wish you all the best on your journey.

Where to Learn More About Dr. Vandana Shiva's Work

To explore Dr Vandana Shiva's inspiring work on environmental sustainability and social justice, visit the Navdanya website at navdanya.org. Founded by Dr Shiva, Navdanya is dedicated to promoting biodiversity, organic farming, and seed sovereignty, providing a platform for transformative education and meaningful action.

Navdanya offers hands-on workshops and learning opportunities covering important topics such as organic farming, eco-feminism, and regenerative agriculture. These workshops give participants the chance to engage directly in sustainable practices, empowering them to contribute to a healthier planet and a fairer food system.

For a deeper understanding of her philosophies, explore Dr. Shiva's extensive collection of books, where she addresses issues of environmental justice, food sovereignty, and the essential role of women in sustainable development. Additionally, her powerful documentary, *The Seeds of Vandana Shiva*, showcases her journey as a tireless advocate for farmers and the environment, offering a compelling insight into her life's work and the global impact of her activism.

Through her writings, workshops, and this documentary, Dr Shiva inspires individuals to be part of creating a future that prioritises ecological balance and social equity. By connecting with Navdanya and engaging with her film, you'll gain a comprehensive view of her mission to build a sustainable and just world.

A Personal Reflection on Our Relationship with Mother Earth

After my conversation with Dr. Vandana Shiva, I reflected on our relationship with the Earth. Her words helped me see that the Earth is not just a resource to be exploited, it is our mother, Mother Earth, who nurtures, provides, and sustains all life. Yet, we've allowed powerful corporations to exploit her, treating the planet with the same disregard that has historically been inflicted upon marginalised communities. Dr Shiva's insights opened my eyes to the situation's urgency—it's time we wake up and take meaningful action.

My research made it clear that Mother Earth is crying out for help. The relentless push for higher production—driven by genetically modified seeds, intensive farming methods, and industrial agriculture—has pushed the planet beyond its natural limits. These technologies were marketed as solutions to crises like famine and drought, but the reality is far more complex. Food quality has declined, prices have risen, and the promises of industrial agriculture have fallen short.

This realisation made me question our current agricultural system. The way forward seems clear: we must return to traditional, respectful farming practices that honour the Earth. Small farmers who work in harmony with the land, using natural methods to grow crops, are the true stewards of the soil and our planet.

Supporting these farmers isn't just about staying healthy, it's about sustaining the Earth for future generations.

Food doesn't just fuel our bodies—it shapes our existence and the world we leave behind. Genetically modified, chemically treated, and industrially produced food alters our health and disrupts natural ecosystems. The choices we make around food today shape the future of our planet, and we cannot take this responsibility lightly.

As I continue on this journey of discovery, I am increasingly aware of the importance of mindfulness in our food choices. Simple, intentional changes—like supporting local farmers, choosing organic and sustainable products, and reconnecting with nature—can significantly impact our food choices. Mother Earth is calling us to restore a respectful and harmonious relationship with her, and we must answer that call.

Reflecting on the Great Reset and Digital Control

Beyond the environment, my conversation with Dr. Shiva sparked deep reflection on the broader changes reshaping our world. The concept of the Great Reset, introduced by the World Economic Forum during the pandemic, was framed as a global plan to rebuild the economy in a more equitable and sustainable way. At first, it seemed promising focused on economic transformation, green energy, and digital innovation. But after diving deeper, I wondered: Who truly benefits from this 'reset'? And who is being left behind?

While the Great Reset claims to promote equity and sustainability, many of the world's largest corporations have significantly benefited from the shifts it has caused. This raised troubling questions for me. The same companies that profit during crises often claim to have the solutions to fix them, creating a cycle of dependency and control. Can we really trust these systems to make the equitable world they promise? Or are they simply reinforcing existing power structures?

The Four Industrial Revolutions

To better understand these changes, I reflected on the Four Industrial Revolutions:

1. The First Industrial Revolution: In the late 1700s, coal and mechanisation transformed industries, laying the groundwork for modern capitalism.

2. The Second Industrial Revolution: By the late 1800s, mass production, assembly lines, and electricity revolutionised industry and communication, reshaping societies.

3. The Third Industrial Revolution: In the late 20th century, computers and the Internet launched us into the digital age and transformed how we live and work.

4. The Fourth Industrial Revolution: Today, we are living through an era marked by the fusion of physical, digital, and biological technologies—AI, robotics, and digital currencies are blurring the lines between our digital and physical worlds.

While these revolutions have brought remarkable progress, they've also introduced new concerns about control and surveillance, particularly in this Fourth Industrial Revolution.

Digital Convenience or Digital Control?

As Dr Shiva pointed out, the rise of FinTech—financial technologies like mobile payments, digital currencies, and online banking—brings both convenience and control. While these tools make life easier, they also track our every move. Each transaction leaves a digital footprint, allowing companies and governments to monitor and influence our financial behaviours.

This leads to a deeper question: Is digital convenience simply a new form of control? How much freedom do we have if every aspect of our lives is digitised and monitored?

Food Control in a Digital World

Dr. Shiva's insights on food control add another layer to this conversation. Today, corporations like Bayer and Corteva control the seeds that farmers rely on. Once farmers could save and replant seeds year after year, but now many are forced to buy new seeds annually from these corporations. This strips farmers of their independence and ties them to corporate-controlled supply chains.

But what happens when food production itself becomes fully digitised? Imagine a future where a few powerful corporations control every step of the food process—from planting to distribution. In such a world, even our access to food could be dictated by corporate interests, turning one of our most basic needs into a controlled commodity.

Who Really Owns Everything?

As I researched further, I realised that many of the corporations benefiting from the Great Reset are owned by the same large financial institutions—BlackRock and Vanguard. These asset management giants hold significant stakes in companies like Amazon, Tesla, Pfizer, and Google, as well as agricultural giants like Bayer and Corteva. With trillions of dollars in assets, they wield immense power over the global economy—and, by extension, over our everyday lives.

This concentration of power raises serious concerns. If a few entities control our food, finances, and technology, how much freedom do we truly have?

A Call to Awareness and Action

We must remain vigilant as we enter the Fourth Industrial Revolution. While the world may seem to be progressing toward greater convenience and efficiency, we must ask: at what cost? Are we unknowingly trading away our freedom for the illusion of convenience?

The Great Reset and the rapid advancements of the Fourth Industrial Revolution are transforming our world. But we have a choice: Will we passively accept these changes or actively shape the future?

After my conversation with Dr. Shiva, I feel more compelled than ever to dig deeper into these issues. I encourage you to do the same. As seekers of wisdom and stewards of the Earth, we must question the systems that seek to control us and take action to protect our freedom, the planet, and future generations.

Reflection Activity:
Our Connection to the Earth

These activities are designed to encourage personal reflection and critical thinking while offering practical steps to engage with the ideas discussed in the conversation with Dr. Vandana Shiva. Through these exercises, you'll explore your relationship with the Earth, the food systems we rely on, and the impacts of corporate control, helping you understand how we can support life on this planet.

Activity 1: Personal Reflection

Journal Prompt: 'Mother Earth as a Nurturer'

Take some time to reflect on Dr. Shiva's metaphor of the Earth as our mother.

- How does this idea resonate with you?

Write down your thoughts about how your daily choices, like the food you eat or the products you buy—affect the Earth.

- Consider small changes you could make to show greater care for the planet.

- Think about how you can nurture and protect the Earth in your daily routine.

Activity 2: Investigate Your Food System

Explore Your Food Choices

Go through your pantry or refrigerator and see where your food comes from.

- Are the ingredients organic?

- Are they locally sourced?

- Or are they from large-scale corporations?

Research a couple of the food brands you regularly buy. Do independent companies own them, or do large corporations control them? Do these companies use sustainable practices?

Food Independence

Reflect on Dr Shiva's ideas about seed control and food sovereignty. How can you take steps towards becoming more independent in your food choices? Here are a few ideas:

- Start growing your own herbs or vegetables

- Shop at farmers' markets to support local growers.

- Reduce reliance on processed foods and focus on whole, unmodified ingredients.

Activity 3: The Digital World and Control

Reflection: Digital Convenience vs Digital Control

Dr Shiva raised concerns about the increasing use of digital tools.

- Make a list of the digital tools you depend on, like mobile payments, online banking, or digital platforms.

- How do these tools impact your privacy and freedom?

- Please take a moment to journal any concerns you have about the balance between convenience and control in this increasingly digital age.

Activity 4: Cash Challenge:

For one week, challenge yourself to only use cash for your daily transactions. Pay for groceries, dining out, transportation, and other necessities with cash instead of using credit cards or digital payment apps.

Reflect on the experience:

- How does it feel to use cash instead of digital payments?

- Did it change your awareness of your spending habits or purchasing decisions?

- What were the reactions of businesses and individuals when you chose to pay with cash?

Activity 5: Connecting with Nature

Spend Time in Nature

Set aside time to walk, hike, or sit in a garden or park. While you're outside, take a moment to reflect on the cycles of life and growth that Dr Shiva mentioned.

- How does spending time in nature make you feel?

- How can you foster a deeper connection with the Earth?

Plant Something

Whether it's an herb in a pot or a small garden, commit to planting something to nourish you and the Earth.

- Reflect on how planting a seed mirrors Dr Shiva's care, growth, and sustainability teachings.

Activity 6: Research and Learning

Further Reading and Research

Choose one of the following topics to research more deeply:

- Seed sovereignty and how it affects food systems.

- The environmental and health impacts of GMOs and industrial agriculture.

- The Great Reset and its implications for our future.

- The role of digital technologies and currencies in the global economy.

Book Recommendations

To dive deeper into the topics discussed by Dr Shiva, pick up one of her books, *Stolen Harvest* or *Oneness vs the 1%*. As you read, take notes on key insights and think about how these ideas can be applied to your life.

Activity 7: Call to Action

Create Your Own Action Plan

After reflecting on everything you've learned from Dr Shiva's conversation, consider how to start living more sustainably.

- Set clear, realistic goals for yourself, like reducing your consumption of processed foods, planting a garden, or choosing to shop locally. Track your progress and celebrate each positive change you make!

Reflection Questions:

- What surprised you the most about Dr Shiva's perspectives on the Earth, food systems, and corporate control?

- How can you incorporate her teachings into your daily habits and choices?

- What actions can you take to raise awareness about these issues within your community?

Concluding Thoughts:

Remember, even small actions can lead to significant change. By reconnecting with the Earth and making mindful decisions, you contribute to a global movement that seeks to honour and protect the planet. Dr Shiva's wisdom reminds us that we are all stewards of the Earth, and it's our responsibility to care for her—for ourselves and future generations.

You and Me

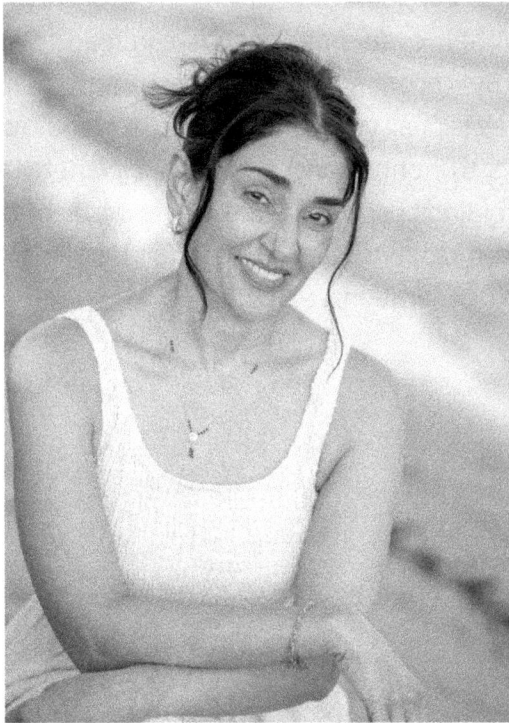

The Seekers of Wisdom and Knowledge

Finding My Place Between Two Worlds

My journey began in 1970 in London. Although I am Indian by heritage, I like to say, 'Indian, made in England, living in Australia.' For me, home is wherever I am in the world. I travel often to visit my aging parents in England, while my husband's parents live in India, making Mother Earth my true home.

My parents came from Gujarat, a small village in Kutch, Bhuj, and moved to London seeking better opportunities. I grew up immersed in a deeply traditional and patriotic Indian culture. Back then, a woman's role was clearly defined: first, she belonged to her father—or, in his absence, to her brother—and later, to her husband.

The expectation was simple back then. It was to get a good education to secure a good marriage. Even the smallest skills, like making the perfectly round chapati, were seen as essential. I remember sneaking into the kitchen just as my father came home, pretending to help—while my sister, the eldest, did most of the actual work. It was my cheeky way of dodging kitchen duties.

From an early age, I was quietly curious about the rules and expectations placed on me. Inside our home, we lived a traditional Indian life—speaking Gujarati, eating home-cooked Indian meals, and watching my mother move gracefully in her sari. But the world outside our door was different. The Western culture I was exposed to presented freedoms and ideas that conflicted with the traditions I had grown up with.

Living between these two worlds was both a gift and a challenge. It gave me the freedom to explore new ways of thinking, but it also left me feeling caught between identities. I wasn't fully at home in either world, always trying to fit into both. In many ways, I was what you might call a 'confused Indian'—navigating the tension between honouring my roots and following my own path.

Too Unclean for the Kitchen

One of my earliest memories is of my mother during her menstrual cycle. She wouldn't enter the kitchen because she was considered 'unclean.' I didn't understand the significance of this ritual. Only later did I realise that what had originally been a way to honour a woman's need for rest had been distorted into something shameful.

Like many households in the 1970s, the human body and menstrual cycle awareness weren't openly discussed in our home. You picked up bits and pieces through friends or maybe at school, but for the most part, you were left to figure things out on your own. There was no gentle introduction, just the deep end of experience waiting for you.

When I got my first period, it felt like the beginning of the end—like I was dying. I remember sitting on the stairs of our old Victorian house, counting how many years I would have to endure this strange, frightening thing called menstruation. The fear of red stains on my nightie haunted me. I hid my bleeding in shame, terrified of being discovered, believing that to be seen would somehow expose me as dirty or defective.

I recall my first experience with severe cramps came after an Indian wedding. The pain overwhelmed me, leaving me curled up in bed, helpless. I had no idea that a simple painkiller could have brought relief—talking about menstruation wasn't something I felt comfortable doing. So, I suffered in silence, unaware that a small tablet of aspirin could have eased my pain.

That moment became a reflection of a deeper pattern that would shape much of my life: enduring pain quietly and without asking for help. It's a belief system I am still working to unlearn to this day—learning that I don't have to carry everything alone, and that asking for help is not a sign of weakness.

Entering Into Womanhood

As I entered my teenage years, I began to see the rigid traditions shaping the lives of young girls in our community. Among Indian families in England, arranged marriages were still the norm, even though India itself had begun to move on. It seemed as though the immigrants who had arrived in the UK during the 1960s and 70s clung even more tightly to their cultural roots, fearing that loosening their grip might mean losing their identity in a foreign land.

I witnessed these customs unfold all around me. Families arranged formal meetings where young men, accompanied by their parents, would visit the homes of prospective brides. Achievements and ambitions were paraded like credentials in a business transaction, but only as a way to enhance marriage prospects. Education, rather than being a path to independence, was seen as an asset to attract a suitable husband. Once married, the girl would leave her family behind and step into her role within her husband's household.

I knew early on that this life wasn't for me. I didn't want my worth tied to how well I could fit into someone else's idea of a 'good wife.' In a quiet act of defiance, I did what was considered unthinkable for a young Indian woman: I started dating an 'Indian bad boy.' Drawn to his mischievous spirit and defiance of tradition, I saw in him a reflection of my own desire to break free from cultural expectations. Every secret moment we spent together felt like a small rebellion, a taste of the freedom I so deeply craved.

In our community, back then, dating wasn't just about exploring a relationship, it came with the implicit promise of marriage. Ending things would not have been a simple breakup; it would have brought shame and judgment upon me and my family. So, I stayed, afraid of the consequences of walking away, even though the relationship began to unravel by my early twenties. At just 20, I found myself married—not because I believed in the relationship, but because I felt trapped by the pressure to marry. Anything seemed better than the shame of being 'left on the shelf' or becoming an outcast in the eyes of the community.

The Dark Night of the Soul

The marriage didn't last. Ending it was one of the hardest decisions I've ever made. Divorce was almost unheard of for Indian women at the time, and my parents treated it like a tragedy. To them, it felt like a death in the family. Their heartbreak weighed heavily on me, and I carried that burden silently, unwilling to add to their pain. But I knew I couldn't stay in a marriage that was slowly breaking me.

Leaving the marriage felt like severing ties not just with my husband but with much of my community. I had to navigate the legal process alone, with no blueprint and little support. At just 23, I was forced to rebuild my life from scratch—isolated, judged, and warned by relatives that I would only attract an older or disabled man now that I was divorced.

In the midst of that darkness, however, I discovered a flicker of light. A few close friends and some relatives, those who quietly admired my courage, offered me support. Their encouragement helped me begin to see that leaving wasn't the end; it was a beginning. That experience sparked a new resolve within me: I would never again let anyone else define my worth or happiness.

Determined to reclaim my independence, I knew I had to leave the familiar confines of London and discover the world on my own terms. That first dark night of the soul marked the beginning of a long journey toward self-discovery. I've since learned that life will present us with many such dark nights, each one forcing us to let go of the person we thought we were and making space for the person we are becoming.

That divorce, painful as it was, set me on a path toward the life I was meant to live. It was the first step in rewriting my story, no longer dictated by cultural expectations, but by my own choices and desires.

A One-Way Ticket to Freedom

In 1996, I made the unthinkable decision to leave behind the life I knew, along with all the cultural expectations that came with it. I bought a one-way ticket to Perth, Australia. A good friend of mine, who was tired of wasting two hours a day in traffic on the North Circular Road, decided to join me. We set off together, each armed with an oversized backpack we'd soon regret. The weight was unbearable. After several months of lugging it around, I downsized my pack to just eight kilos. As I shed the extra weight, I felt as though I was also releasing the burdens of tradition and expectation. For the first time in my life, I felt free. I could do what I wanted, when I wanted—and most exhilarating of all— anywhere in the world.

For a young Indian woman, this was almost scandalous. My parents were terrified, convinced I'd be kidnapped by taxi drivers and sold for my organs. But none of that happened. Instead, I had the time of my life. It was on this journey that the seeker within me truly awakened. I began to let go—not just of cultural expectations but also of my fear of judgment and the belief that I had to fit into a particular mould.

As I travelled through Australia, India, and beyond, I experienced freedom like never before. With each step, I allowed myself to be—free from the pressures of tradition or the need to meet anyone's expectations. Shedding the weight of my old life felt as liberating as reducing my backpack. I wasn't just travelling light; I was letting go of years of conditioning and making space for something new to emerge within me.

This journey wasn't just an escape; it was a return to myself. I discovered that the world was far bigger than I'd imagined, and with it came the realisation that the possibilities for my life were endless. I wasn't defined by the rules I grew up with or by the labels others placed on me. I was free to explore, ask questions, and, most importantly, embrace the unknown.

Starting Over in a Man's World

After a year and a half of travelling, I returned to England, but it quickly became clear that I wasn't the same person anymore. Life in England no longer fit. Soon enough, the urge to leave resurfaced, and in 1999, I moved to Australia, ready to start my career as a financial planner.

Working in finance felt like stepping into the heart of patriarchy. It was a man's world, and being a woman in this industry came with a whole new set of challenges. When I succeeded, my male colleagues would attribute my achievements to my looks, claiming that being a woman made it easier to close deals. But when things didn't go as well, the same colleagues would say I wasn't cut out for the job—claiming I didn't have the mental abilities to understand figures to be a good financial planner. Ridiculous, right? It was a lose-lose situation.

Still, despite the setbacks, things were slowly changing. I persisted, determined to prove my success was not tied to anyone's narrow assumptions. My journey had already taught me that I didn't need to live up to anyone's expectations but my own. I was approaching my mid-30s, and as society so often reminds women, the biological clock's ticking became a constant hum in the background.

But I wasn't ready to settle for just anyone. As much as I knew I wanted a family, I wouldn't compromise my values or rush into something that didn't feel right. Then, as I approached my 36th birthday, I met my husband. It was 2005, and with him, I began a new chapter. For the first time, I allowed myself to surrender my fierce independence and let someone in.

This marked the beginning of my next rite of passage, one that would redefine what independence and partnership truly meant to me.

A Turning Point

The financial crisis of 2008 hit two weeks before my baby was due, and I was made redundant. It wasn't my decision—it felt like a punch to the gut. We had just taken out a mortgage, my husband had launched a new business, and I was suddenly unemployed. I remember the wave of emotions: fear, rejection, and betrayal. What was I going to do with a baby on the way and no income?

But as time passed, I realised that losing my job was a blessing in disguise. It gave me the unexpected opportunity to become a full-time mother, something I likely wouldn't have chosen on my own, given the financial security my career had provided. With the decision made for me, my husband and I agreed that I would stay home with our baby, especially since both of our families lived far away. And so began my journey into motherhood.

Entering Into Motherhood

Becoming a mother was both a shift and a challenging transition. It felt as though my old self had died, and I was stepping into an unfamiliar version of myself. Motherhood, much like menopause, demanded that I let go of what was familiar and embrace the unknown. My baby depended on me entirely, and although I felt unprepared, an instinctive wisdom within me guided the way. Over time, I realised that raising another human being would be the most important and impactful role of my life.

Like all rites of passage, motherhood comes with grief. Every major life transition—whether it's childbirth, parenthood, or menopause—requires us to say goodbye to the person we once were. At first, we don't know who we are becoming, but the new version of ourselves is always greater than what we leave behind. Each loss, though painful, offers a chance to grow, evolve, and love in deeper ways.

The Invisible Work of Motherhood

Stepping fully into the role of a stay-at-home mother wasn't easy. I learned that, despite its importance, motherhood isn't valued the way it should be. Raising a well-rounded generation capable of thriving in today's complex world is one of the most critical jobs, but it's rarely acknowledged. With the rising cost of living, the idea of dedicating yourself entirely to raising children has become increasingly difficult. Mothers are expected to manage careers, parenting, and household responsibilities—often at the expense of their own well-being.

I felt the weight of this pressure at social gatherings when people asked, 'What do you do?' I would lower my head and quietly say, 'I'm just a mum. A housewife.' It felt small, as though it didn't carry the same weight as a professional title. What I didn't realise at the time was that bringing life into the world and nurturing the next generation is one of the most meaningful roles anyone can have.

KPIs for Motherhood

To stay grounded and give myself a sense of accomplishment, I created personal KPIs—Key Performance Indicators—for my days. Every day, I made sure to do a load of laundry, keep the house clean, go to the gym, and prepare dinner. These small routines gave my life structure and purpose, helping me stay present through the chaos of early motherhood.

One of the most important KPIs came from an unexpected place—a tip I read on the back of a nappy box. It suggested reading to your baby three times a day. I made it part of my daily routine, and it became a habit. I didn't know it then, but those moments sparked a love for books in my daughter that continues to this day. It's one of my proudest achievements—knowing that the simple act of reading together not only created a bond but also fostered a lifelong passion for learning.

Making the Most of What We Had

With money tight during those early years, we had to be resourceful. My food budget was just $45 a week, so every Tuesday, I would head to the Victoria Market in search of bargains. My weekly KPI was to host a dinner party—our way of staying social despite our financial constraints. Those gatherings reminded me that life was still happening, even if it looked different from what I had imagined.

Once a month, my husband and I treated ourselves to a night out. We would hire a babysitter and enjoy a meal together for three precious hours. Those evenings felt like pure luxury, and we cherished every moment.

Motherhood Lessons

Things have changed since those early years, but the lessons I learned remain with me. Motherhood taught me resilience, patience, and the value of simplicity. The daily KPIs—the ones no one else saw—were among the most important milestones in my life. They reminded me that the work of raising children, though undervalued by the world, creates the foundation for the future.

Being a mother has shown me that life's most meaningful work often takes place in quiet moments, such as reading bedtime stories, folding laundry, or preparing meals. These seemingly small acts build connections, foster growth, and create a sense of belonging that will stay with our children long after they've grown.

Looking back, those early years of motherhood shaped me as much as they shaped my children. They taught me that the unseen work of raising a family holds unmatched power, and that is no small thing.

Rites of Passage
A Journey into Perimenopause

By my mid-40s, while raising two children under the age of five, I sensed another transition quietly approaching. My body began to shift, and the once-predictable rhythm of my menstrual cycle started to unravel. Irregularities crept in—clots, heavy cramping, and erratic periods that arrived without warning. Along with these physical changes came new cravings. I found myself reaching for sugar and junk food more often, and the weight started to creep on, slowly but steadily.

Then came my first hot flush—unexpected and unforgettable. I was sitting in a bar in Australia, sipping a glass of wine, when a sudden wave of heat surged through me. In an instant, I was drenched in sweat, frantically dabbing my face with a napkin, embarrassed and bewildered by how quickly it hit me. That moment was my wake-up call—my body was speaking loud and clear, and it was time to start listening.

Not long after, anxiety arrived like an uninvited guest. At first, it came quietly, but before long, it lingered every morning. You know that feeling when you open your eyes and the weight of worry is already pressing down on you—before the day has even begun? Simple tasks I had once handled effortlessly—like running errands, driving to new places, or hosting guests—suddenly became overwhelming. Even routine chores that used to be second nature now felt insurmountable, as if they had turned into mountains I didn't know how to climb.

It felt as though my mind and body were speaking a new language—one I hadn't yet learned to interpret. I found myself standing on the edge of an unfamiliar landscape, forced to confront a new kind of challenge: navigating a phase of life without a map. Every step forward felt uncertain as if I were inching my way through the fog, unsure of what lay ahead.

But as unsettling as these changes were, something inside me knew that they were part of a larger process. Just as motherhood had transformed me—leading me through the grief of losing my old self and toward a new identity—so, too, would this next transition. It was another rite of passage, another invitation to release who I had been and make room for the woman I was becoming.

Like every transformation before, this phase required surrender. I had to trust the unknown and allow myself to be shaped by it, even when it felt uncomfortable and disorienting. Every rite of passage carries with it the promise of becoming—of meeting a version of ourselves we have not yet known. And so, I leaned into the uncertainty, trusting that this, too, would guide me toward something meaningful.

Redefining My Perimenopause Journey

As I stepped into my perimenopause journey, I sought wisdom from older women, hoping they could guide me through this transition. But every time I asked them to share their experiences, they would lower their heads in shame, whispering as if we were discussing something forbidden. Their responses reflected a sense of defeat like this was the end of the road. I couldn't accept that. I didn't want my journey to look like that. Surely, life couldn't just stop after menopause. What about everything I had done and everything I still wanted to do?

These conversations sparked my journey into deeper research and discovery. I began seeking out women who had embraced this phase of life and found new meaning in it. But in the midst of these changes, my body and mind felt out of control. Before perimenopause, I might feel anxious for a day or two if something big was happening. Now, the anxiety lingered for weeks, sometimes even months. Hot flushes struck without warning, and I realised I needed to do something drastic to take back control.

That's when I remembered my aunt, who had become a raw vegan and embraced fasting back in 2016. She told me how these lifestyle changes had eased her anxiety and brought her peace. Desperate for relief, I decided to follow her advice. Even though we didn't have the money at the time, I booked myself into a juice fast at the White Lotus Retreats in Byron Bay, hosted by Sarah Foley.

Due to a last-minute cancellation, I was the only guest on the retreat, giving me the rare gift of five days alone. As a mother with young children, uninterrupted time for myself felt like an impossible luxury. I was treated to juices, massages, colonics, and, most importantly, solitude. For the first time in a long while, I could just be.

During that retreat, I stumbled upon a podcast by Dr. Christiane Northrup, and her words planted a powerful seed in my mind. She described menopause as the ultimate wake-up call—a time when a woman unapologetically becomes who she is meant to be and shouts it out loud for the world to hear. Her perspective changed everything for me. This was the path I wanted to follow. Menopause wasn't the end, it was the beginning of something magical.

That retreat marked the start of my journey into self-care and acceptance. It opened the door to learning from other inspiring women, many of whom are featured in this book. Their stories have taught me invaluable lessons and challenged me to view menopause as an invitation to step into the most empowered version of myself.

I hope that through their experiences and insights, you too will be inspired to see menopause as more than just an ending. It's the beginning of the best chapter of your life—a time to embrace who you truly are, unapologetically and without fear.

Embracing the Wonders of Menopause After ten years of research and personal experience, I knew I had to share what I had learnt so others would not have to navigate this journey alone. There is so much more to menopause than physical symptoms—it is a mental and spiritual awakening, a time to confront unresolved issues and explore beliefs we've long buried under life's demands. If we ignore these signs, they will surface in the form of physical discomfort—hot flushes, joint pain, or fatigue—our bodies knocking at the door, asking us to listen. And if we continue to ignore them, those knocks grow louder, sometimes manifesting as illness or disease, signalling that something within us needs healing.

I reached out to Dr. Christiane Northrup, the woman who had sparked this shift in my life. Her groundbreaking work on women's health had helped me see menopause not as an end, but as a powerful beginning. I invited her to be part of this book, and to my surprise, her response came on January 10th, the day after my 54th birthday.

She said yes. Her presence in this book felt like a blessing, an affirmation that I was on the right path.

A Journey of Rebirth

When I began writing this book, I didn't realise I was nearing the end of my perimenopausal years. By the time I completed this book, I had officially entered post-menopause, stepping fully into a new phase of life. Looking back, I see that this book has been both a record of my journey and a reflection of my own rebirth. I am not the same woman I was when I began—I have become the woman I was always meant to be.

Menopause is often misunderstood as an ending, but I've come to see it as a powerful period of gestation. Much like pregnancy, it's a time of inner transformation, when a new self is quietly taking shape, nurtured by wisdom, experience, and the lessons of a lifetime. And with every transformation, there are contractions— moments of discomfort, grief, or challenge. But each contraction has a purpose; it pushes us forward, helping us shed old layers and reveal a truer, freer self.

Rediscovering the Self Beneath the Roles

As I look to the next 30 years, I am filled with excitement and anticipation. I find myself reconnecting with the adventurous spirit I had before I entered womanhood—the girl who questioned everything, sought knowledge, and embraced life with curiosity. That's the woman I want to be again: someone who keeps learning, growing, and evolving, unbound by old expectations or societal roles.

Menopause has given me the freedom to rediscover who I am beneath the roles I have played—the daughter, the mother, the partner, the caretaker. It is an opportunity to peel back those layers and see myself clearly. In this way, menopause is a gift, a chance to return to our core essence, carrying forward only what serves our true selves.

Honouring Cycles and Passing Down Wisdom

One of the greatest joys of this journey has been passing down the wisdom I've gained to my children. I've guided my daughters through their own rites of passage with celebration, not shame. Before their menstrual cycles began, I reminded them: **Remember who you are now, because this is the person you'll reconnect with later in life.**

When their cycles arrived, we celebrated together, marking the occasion with love and support. I want them to understand their bodies and to honour their natural rhythms, just as I've learnt to do. By sharing this knowledge with them, I hope I'm giving them the tools to navigate their own life transitions with confidence, self-respect, and joy.

This respect for cycles has guided me in mothering my daughters and shaped my daily life.

Living in Harmony with Natural Rhythms

Writing this book has taught me the beauty of working in harmony with natural cycles. I began to notice that each day mirrored the seasons: mornings were my 'spring,' a time of creation and focus; afternoons became my 'summer,' a time for sharing ideas and connecting with others; evenings felt like 'autumn,' a time to wind down and reconnect with family; and nights became my 'winter,' a time for rest and renewal.

The same rhythms applied to my months and seasons. With each new moon, I planted the seeds of my intentions. As the moon waxed, I nurtured these ideas, bringing them to life. By the waning moon, I slowed down, reflecting on what I had accomplished and preparing to rest. Just as nature moves through cycles of growth and renewal, I aligned my work and life with these phases, allowing creativity to ebb and flow naturally.

As I embraced these natural rhythms, I discovered a truth that feels important to share wisdom is something we each find for ourselves.

An Invitation to Seek Your Own Wisdom

If you are holding this book in your hands, then you, too, are a seeker of wisdom and knowledge. I encourage you to do your own research, to explore, question, and discover your own truth—whatever resonates and brings you peace. Seek out books, mentors, or communities that inspire you. Do not just take my word for it; true wisdom comes from seeking knowledge and experiencing life firsthand.

The incredible women whose stories have shaped this book taught me that there's power in honouring your experiences and turning them into something meaningful. They are reshaping humanity by living courageously, unapologetically, and with a deep respect for the natural cycles of life. Take inspiration from them, but trust your own journey. Seek out what feels right for you, and let your path unfold as it's meant to.

Embrace the New Life Waiting to Be Born

Menopause, like any birth, comes with contractions. There will be moments of discomfort, of grief for the woman you once were, and times when the changes feel overwhelming. But each contraction has a purpose; it is guiding you toward the life waiting to be born. Just as labour brings forth new life, menopause brings forth a new chapter—one where you have the freedom to be exactly who you are, unapologetically and joyfully.

So, here's my invitation to you: explore what brings you joy, and make it a part of your life. Use this time to reconnect with your core self and celebrate every step of the way. Like the cycles of nature, every season of life brings its own gifts, each one waiting to be discovered.

This is your season to bloom, to shed what no longer serves you, and to nurture what is ready to grow. Embrace this time of gestation, this journey of rebirth, and trust that you are becoming the woman you were always meant to be.

The Best

Is

Yet to Come

Shavita Kotak
Seven Wonders of Menopause

Where to Learn More About Shavita Kotak

Shavita Kotak is a seeker of wisdom and knowledge, a journey that has taken her around the world to immerse herself in ancient teachings. She has spent long periods of time learning from ashrams in India, participating in silent Vipassana retreats, and engaging in extended fasting to connect deeply with her soul. Since 2003, Shavita has been teaching and practising yoga, using her personal experiences to guide and inspire others.

In addition, Shavita facilitates sound healing as a powerful tool to help others manage the stresses of today's world and connect deeply within themselves. She also leads women's circles, creating sacred spaces for women to share, grow, and support each other on their transformative journeys.

Shavita also hosts a YouTube channel with over 400 classes on meditation, yoga, Pilates, and self-care practices, ranging from 10 minutes to an hour. These offerings provide accessible resources for individuals seeking well-being and inner peace.

For more information about Shavita's offerings, events, and workshops, visit her website at shivitakotak.com. You can also follow her on social media, where she shares her insights and wisdom about the spiritual journey of menopause and beyond. Through her work, Shavita inspires others to embrace transformation with courage, grace, and intention.

Reflection Activity

Tips for Thriving Through Perimenopause and Beyond

Tip 1: Start Early: Prepare in Your Late 30s or Early 40s

Begin building a solid self-care routine long before menopause starts. Take care of your body and mind through:

- **Eating well:** Nourish yourself with wholesome foods.

- **Exercise:** Move your body regularly in ways that feel good.

- **Silence & meditation:** Take time daily for quiet moments to reset and reflect.

Tip 2: Embrace Aging - Let Go of Youth-Centered Pressure

Our culture idolises youth, but trying to hold onto it can drain your energy. Release the fear of aging. Instead:

- **Celebrate every stage of life** for the wisdom it brings.

- Focus on **nurturing your mind, body, and spirit** rather than chasing youth.

- **Prioritise joy** - be happy with where you are now.

Tip 3: Evaluate Relationships — Choose Wisely

- Pay attention to how your interactions affect you:

- **Ask yourself:** After spending time with someone, do I feel uplifted or drained?

- **Nurture relationships** that inspire and energise you.

- Gradually **let go of toxic connections** that no longer serve you.

Tip 4: Fast to Reset and Recenter

Fasting can be a powerful tool to help you feel grounded during perimenopause.

- Even **short fasts of 2-3 days** can provide mental clarity and physical renewal.

- **Longer fasts of 5+ days** offer a deep reset and are great for reconnecting with yourself.

Tip 5: Build Your 'No' Muscle — Speak Your Truth

Saying no is a powerful act of self-care. If you say yes to others when you mean no, you say no to yourself.

- **Start small:** Practice saying no even when it feels uncomfortable.

- Each time you say no, you **strengthen your ability** to honour your boundaries.

This will **build confidence** over time, helping you protect your energy.

Tip 6: Create a Supportive Community

Surround yourself with other women—especially postmenopausal women—who understand this transition.

- **Find a community** that can hold space for you without trying to fix or solve everything.

- These women can offer support, wisdom, and a safe space to process your experiences.

Remember: No one can do the inner work for you, but being held in love and support can make the journey easier.

Tip 7: Enjoy This New Chapter – Dance with Life

Perimenopause and menopause are not endings; they are beginnings. Approach this time with curiosity and joy.

- **Sing and dance with the universe** — let life guide you in unfolding what's next.

This is an **exciting time to reconnect** with who you truly are. Embrace it fully.

Closing Thoughts: Embrace the Possibilities

This chapter of life is an invitation—a chance to shed old layers, honour your body's wisdom, and step boldly into who you are meant to be. It's a time to let go of societal expectations and create a life that aligns with your truest self. Yes, challenges will arise, but within them lies the power to transform.

Remember: the work of this journey is yours alone, but you don't have to walk it in isolation. Surround yourself with a circle of supportive women, build nourishing relationships, and seek joy in the small moments. Treat this time as sacred—a season to reflect, renew, and celebrate all that you are becoming.

The beauty of menopause isn't just in surviving it, but in thriving within it. This isn't the end—it's the beginning of a vibrant new chapter filled with possibilities waiting to unfold. So take the universe's hand, dance through the changes, and embrace this time as the powerful transformation it was always meant to be. The best is yet to come.

The Dance of Becoming

This is not the end—oh no, my friend,
It's the start of a chapter where limits transcend.
A time to release what no longer must stay,
To shed old layers and be bold on your way.

The rhythms have shifted, your body now speaks,
With whispers and heatwaves, it nudges, it peaks.
It's calling you inward, to pause and reflect,
To honour the self you've so often neglect.

The world may say youth is the treasure to hold,
But wisdom, dear one, is your gift of pure gold.
Each wrinkle, each scar, a story well-told,
A badge of a life lived fearless and bold.

So dance with the seasons, flow with the moon,
Plant seeds in darkness—they'll flourish soon.
Embrace every phase—the spring and the fall,
For each has a beauty, a purpose, a call.

Say no when it's needed, say yes to your soul,
Build boundaries like bridges, make yourself whole.
Find joy in your circle, in women who share,
In spaces of love where they hold you with care.

This is your moment—don't shrink, but expand,
Take life by the heart and the universe's hand.
The best is before you, unknown and bright,
Your song is still playing—so dance through the night.

For within every change, there's magic to find,
A spark that ignites both the heart and the mind.
This is your awakening, your time to rise—
An endless horizon beneath open skies.

Appendix 1

Navigating Menopause Together – A Partner's Guide

Supporting your partner through menopause can be a new experience, but it's also an opportunity for both of you to grow and deepen your relationship. Menopause involves more than physical changes—it's an emotional and spiritual transformation. By understanding the journey and showing empathy, you can nurture your bond and discover new ways to connect. This guide offers practical tips, grounded in clinical knowledge and relational wisdom, to help you support your partner—and yourself—during this significant life transition.

1. Learn the Basics

Menopause has three main phases:

Perimenopause: The body begins to adjust, with fluctuating hormones causing symptoms like mood changes and irregular cycles.

Menopause: Officially marked by 12 consecutive months without a period, signalling the end of reproductive years.

Post-menopause: Symptoms may ease, and it becomes a time to explore new opportunities for personal growth and relationship renewal.

Tip: Educate yourself. Books like *The Wisdom of Menopause* by Dr. Christiane Northrup provide both medical and emotional insights, helping you understand her experience and make her feel seen and supported.

2. Patience Over Perfection (Mood Swings)

Mood swings are part of the process, driven by fluctuating hormone levels and emotional adjustments. They aren't about you—they reflect what's happening within her.

Tip: Offer empathy with simple words like, 'I'm here for you.' Listening without judgment is often more helpful than offering solutions. Your patience will go a long way during this time of change.

3. Support Her Self-Care

This is a time when she may need to focus more on herself and explore self-care practices that nurture her physically, emotionally, and spiritually. Your support matters.

Tip: Create space for her to engage in activities like yoga, meditation, or journaling. Join her on walks or other relaxing activities to show that you care about her well-being.

4. Stay Cool, Literally (Hot Flushes & Fatigue)

Hot flushes, night sweats, and fatigue can make daily life challenging. Simple environmental changes can make a big difference.

Tip: Keep the bedroom cool with breathable bedding, fans, or open windows. If she needs extra rest, encourage it without guilt—it's part of her body's healing process.

5. Rediscovering Intimacy Together (Libido & Connection)

Menopause can change physical intimacy, but it's also a time to explore deeper emotional connections. This shift can open new opportunities for bonding in different ways.

Tip: Be patient and explore non-sexual intimacy— such as cuddling, holding hands, or sharing quiet moments. Open communication about what feels good for both of you is essential.

6. Make Health a Team Effort

With menopause comes an increased focus on health—both for her and for you. Physical activity, healthy eating, and wellness routines can support both of you.

Tip: Plan healthy meals together, go on walks, or explore new fitness activities as a couple. Wellness can be a shared goal, not just her responsibility.

7. Celebrate Her Strength

Menopause marks the beginning of a powerful new phase in her life. Acknowledging the strength it takes to navigate this transition will deepen your connection.

Tip: Recognise her resilience. Let her know you see the wisdom she is stepping into and celebrate this phase of her life as a time of growth and renewal.

8. Take Care of Yourself Too

Supporting your partner during menopause can be emotionally demanding. You need to take care of your well-being to show up as your best self.

Tip: Find activities that recharge you, whether that's time with friends, exercise, or mindfulness practices. Having your own support system ensures you can stay present and patient.

9. Open Communication – How to Start the Conversation

Talking about menopause can feel daunting, but open communication helps prevent misunderstandings. It builds trust and ensures both of you feel supported.

Tip: Ask questions like:

- 'How can I support you right now?'

- 'What's been on your mind lately?'

These conversations help her feel heard and let her know you're invested in her well-being.

10. Embrace the Change Together

Menopause isn't just her journey—it's an opportunity for you to rediscover each other and grow together. With patience, curiosity, and love, this phase can deepen your connection and create new opportunities for joy.

Tip: See menopause as a rebirth—not only for her but for your relationship. This is a time to embrace the future together and create new ways of being.

Final Thoughts

Menopause is a significant transition—for her, for you, and for your relationship. The most important thing you can do is be present, patient, and willing to grow together. With understanding and empathy, this transition becomes an opportunity to build a stronger relationship and embrace a deeper, more meaningful connection.

Appendix 2

Empower Your Care – Key Questions to Ask Your Doctor During Menopause

Navigating menopause requires more than just symptom management—it's an opportunity to take charge of your health with the right support. Asking thoughtful questions at your doctor's visit ensures you receive care that addresses your symptoms, lifestyle, mental well-being, and long-term goals. This guide will help you advocate for yourself and find your desired healthcare partner.

Before Your Appointment

- **Prepare a List:** To stay organised, write down your symptoms, questions, and concerns.

- **Track Your Symptoms:** Keep a journal to identify patterns like hot flushes, mood changes, or sleep issues.

- **Bring Your Medical History:** If this is your first time with a new provider, bring relevant medical records to ensure seamless care.

1. What key health risks should I focus on during menopause?

- **Why:** Menopause can increase the risk of osteoporosis, heart disease, and metabolic changes. Addressing these risks early helps prevent complications and promotes long-term well-being.

2. How will my diet, exercise, and lifestyle impact my symptoms and long-term health?

- **Why:** Nutrition, physical activity, and stress management can reduce the intensity of menopause symptoms and improve overall health. If your doctor overlooks lifestyle adjustments, it may be a sign that their approach is too narrow.

3. What non-medical approaches do you recommend to manage my symptoms?

- **Why:** Complementary therapies like yoga, meditation, or acupuncture can provide relief and support well-being alongside traditional treatments. A good doctor will consider all options.

4. What are the potential side effects and alternatives if medication is needed?

- **Why:** Hormone replacement therapy (HRT) and other medications come with benefits and risks. Understanding your options helps you make informed decisions about what's best for you.

5. How can we work together to create a long-term health plan?

- **Why:** Menopause is an ongoing journey; your care should evolve with your needs. A collaborative plan ensures you get the right support every step of the way.

6. Do you stay current with the latest menopause research and treatments?

- **Why:** Menopause care evolves, and a good doctor keeps up with new research and treatment guidelines to provide you with the most up-to-date options.

7. How can I improve my emotional and mental well-being during this transition?

- **Why:** Menopause can bring emotional changes, including mood swings and anxiety. A healthcare provider who acknowledges this aspect will offer a more holistic approach to care.

8. How can I improve sleep, energy, and stress management?

- **Why:** Poor sleep and low energy are common symptoms of menopause. Your doctor should offer solutions beyond medication, like relaxation techniques or lifestyle changes, to help you manage these challenges.

9. Can you recommend specialists or resources for additional support?

- **Why:** You may benefit from seeing other professionals, such as a nutritionist, physical therapist, or counsellor. Your doctor should have a network of referrals to ensure you receive the right support.

Red Flags to Watch For

- **The doctor only prescribes medication without discussing lifestyle changes.**

- **Why This Matters:** A doctor who overlooks the role of diet, exercise, or stress management may not provide the holistic care you need. Lifestyle factors play a crucial role in menopause management, and overlooking them can lead to incomplete care.

- **What to Do:** If your doctor focuses solely on medication, say: **'I'd like to explore lifestyle changes alongside medication—how can we approach this together?'**

Final Tip: Trust Your Instincts

Your relationship with your doctor should feel like a partnership where your concerns are heard, and your well-being is prioritised. If your doctor dismisses your questions or overlooks important aspects of your health, it may be time to seek a new provider. **Your health journey is in your hands—ask boldly, trust your instincts, and embrace the wisdom this phase offers.**

Conclusion

Menopause is an opportunity to realign your health, build positive habits, and confidently embrace this new chapter. Asking these thoughtful questions will help you receive the care you deserve and ensure you have a healthcare partner who supports your long-term well-being.

Appendix 3

Menopause Symptoms and Their Spiritual Messages

The journey through menopause is both physical and spiritual. Each symptom can be seen as a contraction—just like in childbirth—signalling the birth of a new self. Rather than viewing these experiences as obstacles, we can understand them as opportunities for healing and renewal. This appendix offers insights into both the physical effects of menopause and their deeper spiritual meanings, empowering you to navigate this transition with greater awareness.

Please note: These spiritual interpretations are intended as one possible perspective to encourage self-reflection and healing. Each individual's experience of menopause is unique, and this appendix offers insights that may or may not resonate with all readers. Consider pairing these reflections with self-care practices that support physical and emotional well-being during menopause.

Hot Flushes and Night Sweats

- **Meaning**: Purification through fire, burning away old patterns and emotional baggage to create space for inner clarity and strength.

- **Physical Impact**: Sudden heat waves, often accompanied by sweating, especially at night.

Mood Swings

- **Meaning**: An invitation to confront and release buried emotions, leading to greater emotional balance and personal growth.

- **Physical Impact**: Intense emotional fluctuations, often challenging to predict.

Vaginal Dryness

- **Meaning**: A call to reconnect with your inner creativity and intimacy in new ways.

- **Physical Impact**: Reduced lubrication, sometimes leading to discomfort.

Sleep Disturbances

- **Meaning**: A signal to reflect on life rhythms and practice deeper self-care.

- **Physical Impact**: Difficulty falling or staying asleep, resulting in fatigue.

Decreased Libido

- **Meaning**: An opportunity to explore passion beyond the physical and reconnect with activities that spark joy.

- **Physical Impact**: A noticeable drop in sexual desire.

Weight Gain

- **Meaning**: An invitation to release emotional burdens and embrace self-acceptance.

- **Physical Impact**: Increased body weight, particularly around the abdomen.

Thinning Hair and Dry Skin

- **Meaning**: A reminder to shed old identities and embrace inner beauty.

- **Physical Impact**: Loss of hair density and reduced skin elasticity.

Brain Fog and Cognitive Changes

- **Meaning**: A chance to live more mindfully, releasing outdated thought patterns.

- **Physical Impact**: Forgetfulness and difficulty concentrating.

Digestive Issues

- **Meaning**: A signal to release emotional tension and align with inner peace.

- **Physical Impact**: Bloating, constipation, or discomfort.

Joint Pain and Stiffness

- **Meaning**: Encourages flexibility—both physically and emotionally—in life transitions.

- **Physical Impact**: Pain or stiffness, often limiting movement.

Urinary Changes

- **Meaning**: A call to let go of emotional toxins and embrace life's flow.

- **Physical Impact**: Increased frequency or urgency to urinate, sometimes accompanied by discomfort.

Itchy Skin

- **Meaning**: Represents the discomfort of shedding old identities to reveal a more authentic self.

- **Physical Impact**: Persistent itching or skin sensitivity.

Frozen Shoulder (Adhesive Capsulitis)

- **Meaning**: A sign to release burdens and welcome support and new possibilities.

- **Physical Impact**: Pain and restricted movement in the shoulder joint, often due to inflammation.

Loss of Bone Density

- **Meaning**: Encourages grounding practices that build emotional and spiritual resilience.

- **Physical Impact**: Reduced bone strength, increasing fracture risk.

Memory Lapses

- **Meaning**: A chance to clear mental clutter and focus on what matters now.

- **Physical Impact**: Temporary forgetfulness or mental blankness.

Conclusion

Menopause is not just a physical experience—it is an invitation to step into a new, empowered version of yourself. Each symptom serves as a messenger, guiding you through a process of renewal, just as contractions lead to the birth of new life. With every wave of discomfort, you are moving closer to your most authentic self, ready to embrace this new chapter with courage, curiosity, and grace. Remember, this journey is yours to navigate with compassion for yourself and trust in your inner strength.

Bibliography

Chapter 1 - Dr. Gladys McGarey

Glossary of Terms

American Holistic Medical Association (AHMA)
An organisation founded in 1978 by Dr. Gladys McGarey and colleagues to support holistic and integrative healthcare, blending traditional and alternative medical practices. The AHMA emphasises whole-person health—addressing wellness's physical, mental, and spiritual aspects.

Dominion vs. Domination
Dr. McGarey distinguishes between 'dominion,' which means responsible stewardship over the Earth, and 'domination,' which implies control and exploitation. Her concept aligns with environmental care philosophies that advocate for a respectful relationship with the natural world.

Geriatric Care
Medical and support services are specifically tailored for the elderly. Dr. McGarey highlights ethical concerns in eldercare, contrasting compassionate, patient-focused models with profit-driven approaches that may overlook the well-being of seniors.

The Five L's
Dr McGarey's guiding life philosophy—Life, Love, Laughter, Labour, and Listening—emphasises a holistic approach to well-being:

- **Life**: Embracing vitality and purpose at every life stage.

- **Love**: Cultivating kindness, compassion, and connection.

- **Laughter**: Recognising the healing power of joy and humour.

- **Labour**: Meaningful work that contributes to one's purpose.

- **Listening**: Practising empathetic listening to oneself and others.

Holistic Medicine

A healthcare approach that considers the entire person—mind, body, and spirit—rather than just treating symptoms. This concept is foundational to Dr McGarey's work, as she advocates for integrated health practices that address all aspects of a person's well-being.

Loneliness and Isolation in Elder Care

Dr McGarey addresses the issue of isolation among the elderly, describing how it negatively impacts physical and mental health. She argues that loneliness is a significant health risk for seniors, comparable to chronic illnesses.

Social Determinants of Health

There are non-medical factors that impact health, such as socioeconomic status, social connections, and access to healthcare. Dr. McGarey advocates for an eldercare model that considers these factors, promoting community-based support over institutionalisation.

Life Transitions

The major phases of life, such as menopause and aging, are considered opportunities for growth and renewal by Dr. McGarey. These transitions are considered spiritual and physical passages, inviting reflection and adaptation.

References

Books by Dr. Gladys McGarey:

- **McGarey, Gladys.** *The Well-Lived Life*. Self-published, 2023.

- o   This book introduces the concept of the 'Five L's' – Love, Laughter, Labor, Listening, and Legacy – as a framework for living a meaningful life.

- **McGarey, Gladys.** *The Physician Within You.* Self-published, 1995.

  - o   This book emphasises holistic medicine and the importance of addressing physical, emotional, and spiritual health in healing practices.

- **McGarey, Gladys.** *Living Medicine.* Self-published, 2010.

  - o   A reflection on life transitions and the role of resilience, adaptability, and purpose in navigating change.

Supporting Works:

- **American Holistic Medical Association** (AHMA). *Our Mission.* Available at: https://www.americanholistichealth.org.

  - o   AHMA's mission to integrate holistic principles into healthcare aligns with Dr. McGarey's advocacy for holistic medicine.

- **Orr, David.** *Earth in Mind: On Education, Environment, and the Human Prospect.* Island Press, 1994.

  - o   Discusses the principles of 'dominion versus domination,' reinforcing Dr. McGarey's perspectives on balanced living.

- **Leopold, Aldo.** *A Sand County Almanac: And Sketches Here and There.* Oxford University Press, 1949.

  - o   Offers insights into harmonious living with nature, complementing the philosophies in Dr. McGarey's work.

- **National Institute on Aging** (NIA). *Social Isolation and Loneliness in Older People*. National Institutes of Health, 2019.

    o Addresses the impact of loneliness and isolation in elder care, a critical aspect of Dr. McGarey's reflections on community and connection.

- **Global Market Insights**. *Geriatric Care Services Market Forecast*. 2021.

    o Provides data on geriatric care services, contextualising Dr. McGarey's discussions on aging and healthcare.

- **Harvard Health Publishing.** *Strategies for Staying Healthy as You Age.'*2019.

    o Offers practical strategies for healthy aging, supporting Dr. McGarey's holistic approach to elder care.

- **World Health Organisation** (WHO). *World Report on Ageing and Health.'*2015.

    o Explores social determinants of health, echoing themes in Dr. McGarey's advocacy for community-focused healthcare.

Chapter 2 - Ibu Robin Lim

Glossary of Terms

Placenta
The placenta is an organ that forms in the uterus during pregnancy, essential for transferring oxygen and nutrients from the mother to the baby. In many cultures, including those in Bali and the Philippines, the placenta is considered sacred, symbolising life and continuity. Following birth, it is often honoured with special rituals or ceremonies.

Delayed Cord Clamping
A birthing practice in which the umbilical cord is left uncut for several minutes after birth, allowing continued blood flow from the placenta to the baby. This practice is believed to enhance newborn iron levels and overall health. At Bumi Sehat, the clinic founded by Ibu Robin Lim, delayed cord clamping is a standard practice, supporting newborn health and promoting bonding between mother and child.

Lotus Birth
A method where the umbilical cord remains uncut, allowing the placenta to naturally detach from the baby over several days. This practice is thought to provide both physical and spiritual benefits, easing the baby's transition into life outside the womb. Ibu Robin Lim supports Lotus Birth as part of a gentle, holistic birth experience at Bumi Sehat.

Full Lotus Birth
A type of Lotus Birth where the umbilical cord and placenta stay attached until they naturally separate. To preserve the placenta during this time, it is typically salted, wrapped in cloth, and kept near the newborn. This approach respects the natural bond between mother, baby, and placenta, a practice embraced at Bumi Sehat.

Guardian Angel (Placenta)
In Balinese culture, the placenta is revered as a 'guardian angel' for the child, offering lifelong spiritual protection. Often buried ceremonially, the placenta represents a lasting connection to the individual and is regarded with profound respect.

Bumi Sehat Foundation
An Indonesian-based non-profit organisation founded by Ibu Robin Lim. Bumi Sehat provides free, respectful maternal and neonatal care, merging traditional birthing practices with modern medical insights. Its mission is to support gentle, culturally attuned birth practices that benefit mothers and babies alike.

Cord Blood
The blood left in the umbilical cord and placenta after birth,

rich in stem cells valuable for medical treatments. In conventional settings, cord blood is often collected for storage, but in natural birthing practices like Lotus Birth, it remains with the newborn, symbolising a commitment to a holistic philosophy of non-separation.

References

Books by Ibu Robin Lim:

- **Lim, Ibu Robin.** *The Placenta: The Forgotten Chakra.* Self-published, 2003.

  o This book explores the role of the placenta beyond its biological function, presenting it as a connector of life and worthy of cultural reverence. She encourages readers to appreciate the placenta as a sacred entity in the birthing process.

Supporting Works:

- **World Health Organisation** (WHO). *Delayed Cord Clamping and Cutting in Newborns.* Available at: https://www.who.int.

  o WHO's guidelines emphasise the health benefits of delayed cord clamping, a practice that aligns with Bumi Sehat's birthing protocols to support bonding and neonatal health.

- **Roshana, Shivam.** *Lotus Birth.* Self-published, 2001.

  o This work examines the practice and benefits of Lotus Birth, advocating a holistic approach to bonding that has lasting effects on child and maternal well-being.

- **South China Morning Post.** *Demand for Hman Placentas in China and the United States.'* Available at: https://www.scmp.com.

  o This article investigates the cultural and commercial uses of the placenta, focusing on its perceived value in traditional medicine across various societies.

- **Parvati Baker, Jeannine**. *Prenatal Yoga and Natural Childbirth*. Self-published, 1986.

  o A key influence on holistic birthing advocates like Ibu Robin Lim, this book promotes natural childbirth and gentle transition practices, including Lotus Birth, as part of a movement towards sacred, intentional birth experiences.

Chapter 3 - Alexandra Pope

Glossary of Terms

Menstrual Cycle Awareness (MCA)
The practice of observing and tracking the physical, emotional, and mental changes throughout the menstrual cycle. By tuning into these natural rhythms, women can connect more deeply with their body's phases, fostering self-awareness, empowerment, and alignment with their inner needs.

Menstruality
A term that encompasses the full journey of a woman's life stages related to the menstrual cycle, including menarche (first menstruation), the monthly cycle, ovulation, pre-menstruum, and menopause. Alexandra Pope emphasises menstruality as a lifelong source of feminine wisdom and personal insight.

The Quickening
A term used by Alexandra Pope to describe the period leading up to menopause, often marked by heightened physical and emotional shifts. This time is viewed as a preparatory phase, guiding women to release what no longer serves them as they transition towards menopause.

Cyclical Consciousness
An awareness of the menstrual cycle's stages and their impact

on energy, mood, and mental clarity. Alexandra encourages women to embrace cyclical consciousness to better align daily activities with their natural rhythms, enhancing physical, mental, and emotional well-being.

Yin Yoga
A slow, gentle form of yoga where postures are held for extended periods, helping to release tension and promote calm. Alexandra Pope recommends Yin Yoga as a practice to support the menstrual cycle, especially during menstruation, for its grounding effects on both body and mind.

Hormonal Contraception
Medications, such as the contraceptive pill, that adjust a woman's hormone levels to prevent pregnancy. Alexandra examines the effects of hormonal contraceptives on intuition, emotional health, and partner preferences, encouraging women to make informed choices that align with their natural cycles.

Menarche
The first menstruation in a young woman's life, marking the beginning of reproductive capability. Alexandra describes menarche as an important rite of passage that shapes a woman's relationship with her body and her menstrual cycle, and she advocates for supportive education around this milestone.

Ovulation
The phase of the menstrual cycle when an egg is released from the ovary, generally associated with peak fertility. Ovulation often brings an increase in energy, confidence, and social engagement, and is a time when women are encouraged to harness this outward-facing energy.

Pre-menstruum
The phase just before menstruation, frequently marked by emotional sensitivity, introspection, and sometimes an intensification of the 'Inner Critic.' Alexandra suggests that this period is an opportunity for rest, self-reflection, and clarity, allowing women to address unresolved issues.

Inner Seasons
A metaphor for the phases of the menstrual cycle, where each phase is likened to a season: menstruation as winter, ovulation as summer, and so forth. This concept helps women understand the distinct energies present throughout the cycle and apply this awareness to enhance their well-being.

Inner Critic
An intensified self-reflective voice often experienced during the pre-menstruum phase. Alexandra regards the Inner Critic as both a challenge and a guide for growth, urging women to understand this inner dialogue as an opportunity for self-improvement.

Psychotherapy
A therapeutic practice involving conversation between a therapist and a client, aimed at fostering mental health and emotional well-being. Alexandra's background in psychotherapy informs her menstruality work, promoting a compassionate, insightful approach to understanding the mind-body connection.

References

Books by Alexandra Pope:

- **Pope, Alexandra, and Sjanie Hugo Wurlitzer.** *Wild Power: Discover the Magic of Your Menstrual Cycle and Awaken the Feminine Path to Power*. Hay House, 2017.

    o   This book offers a comprehensive guide to Menstrual Cycle Awareness (MCA), encouraging readers to discover the wisdom inherent in each phase. Alexandra and Sjanie emphasise how connecting with natural rhythms can bring practical and spiritual benefits.

- **Pope, Alexandra, and Sjanie Hugo Wurlitzer.** *Wise Power: Discover the Liberating Power of Menopause to Awaken Authority, Purpose, and Belonging*. Hay House, 2022.

- o An exploration of menopause as a journey of transformation, positioning this phase as a time for self-discovery, empowerment, and purpose. Alexandra redefines menopause as an awakening to inner authority and strength.

Supporting Works:

- **Hillard, P. J. A.** *Menstrual Suppression: Current Perspectives.* International Journal of Women's Health, vol. 6, 2014, pp. 631–637.

  - o This article examines the effects of menstrual suppression on psychological and physical health, supporting Alexandra's exploration of how hormonal contraception affects women's cycles and intuition.

- **Roberts, S. C., et al.** *Relationship Satisfaction and Outcome in Women Who Meet Their Partner While Using Oral Contraception.* Proceedings of the Royal Society B: Biological Sciences, vol. 279, no. 1732, 2012, pp. 1430–1436.

  - o This study investigates how hormonal contraception influences partner choice and relationship satisfaction, reinforcing Alexandra's observations on how hormonal shifts can affect attraction and compatibility.

- **Guttmacher Institute.** *Contraceptive Use in the United States.* Guttmacher Institute, 2022.

  - o Provides context on the prevalence of hormonal contraceptive use and its long-term effects, offering background for Alexandra's reflections on contraceptive impacts on health and self-awareness.

Organisational References:

- **The Red School** (Founded by Alexandra Pope and Sjanie Hugo Wurlitzer).

o   A UK-based organisation dedicated to teaching Menstrual Cycle Awareness and menstruality through courses, workshops, and resources. Red School advocates for greater menstrual education and body literacy, supporting Alexandra's work in the field of cyclical consciousness.

Chapter 4 - Jane Hardwicke Collings

Glossary of Terms

Shamanic Womancraft
A spiritual and healing practice founded by Jane Hardwicke Collings that combines shamanic principles with feminine wisdom. It honours life's transitions—such as menstruation, childbirth, and menopause—as sacred rites of passage, encouraging women to connect with their natural cycles and embrace personal growth.

Patriarchal Culture
A social structure where men hold primary authority, often shaping societal norms and healthcare in ways that limit women's autonomy. Jane critiques this structure, particularly in maternity care, and advocates for birthing practices that empower women rather than undermine them.

Midwifery
The practice of supporting women through pregnancy and childbirth, traditionally centred on women's needs. Jane advocates for a return to compassionate, holistic midwifery that honours the mother's autonomy and choices, counteracting the more medicalised approaches she views as impersonal and interventionist.

Birth Trauma
Emotional or physical distress resulting from challenging or disempowering childbirth experiences. Often due to unnecessary interventions, birth trauma can impact both mother and child. Jane highlights the importance of healing from such trauma to ensure emotional well-being and advocates for respectful, supportive birthing practices.

Matriarchal Societies
Ancient social structures where women played central roles in decision-making, cultural continuity, and connection to natural cycles. Jane's teachings are inspired by these societies, promoting a revival of matriarchal values in contemporary life, particularly in how women approach childbirth and community.

Hygieia Health
A non-profit organisation co-founded by Jane during the COVID-19 pandemic, focusing on awareness of birth trauma and maternal healing. The foundation's community, 'Mamatoto' (Swahili for 'Motherbaby'), offers resources and support, reflecting Jane's belief in community-centred maternal care.

Herstory
A term coined by Jane to describe history from a female perspective, emphasising women's experiences and ancestral wisdom. In her work *Herstory*, Jane recounts the evolution of patriarchal societies but also celebrates the endurance and strength of feminine wisdom.

Rites of Passage
Ceremonies or rituals marking significant life transitions, such as menarche, motherhood, and menopause. Jane encourages viewing these transitions as sacred opportunities for personal and spiritual growth.

The Red Thread
A metaphor used by Jane to describe the maternal lineage and intergenerational connections passed down through DNA and shared experiences. This concept suggests that both trauma and resilience are inherited, and that healing in one generation can positively impact those that follow.

Ancestral Healing
A process of healing intergenerational trauma, often through acknowledging and processing past wounds. In her teachings, Jane encourages ancestral healing as a way for women to free themselves and future generations from cycles of inherited pain, thus strengthening the maternal lineage.

Womb Wisdom

The intuitive and spiritual knowledge that Jane believes women can access by connecting with their menstrual and reproductive cycles. Womb wisdom encompasses the insights and guidance that come from honouring one's feminine body and its rhythms as sacred.

Sacred Feminine

A spiritual concept that values qualities traditionally associated with femininity—such as intuition, nurturing, creativity, and connection to natural cycles. Jane's work advocates reclaiming the Sacred Feminine as an integral part of women's identities and lives.

Sisterhood Circles

Supportive gatherings where women come together to share experiences, stories, and healing practices. Jane promotes Sisterhood Circles as part of her Shamanic Womancraft approach, creating spaces for women to honour rites of passage, connect with each other, and foster community-based healing.

Dark Goddess

An archetype representing the inner force that brings about necessary transformation. Jane encourages engaging with the 'dark goddess' within as a way to confront and heal unresolved aspects of oneself, tapping into the power that comes from embracing the unknown.

References

Books by Jane Hardwicke Collings:

- **Hardwicke Collings, Jane.** *Blood Rites: The Spiritual Practice of Menstruation*. Self-published, 2005.

    o This book invites readers to view menstruation as a sacred, empowering part of feminine wisdom, encouraging a deeper connection with the cycles of life.

- **Hardwicke Collings, Jane.** *Ten Moons: The Inner Journey of Pregnancy*. Self-published, 2012.

- Explores pregnancy as a journey of personal and spiritual growth, urging women to connect with ancestral wisdom and transformative growth through the birthing experience.

- **Hardwicke Collings,** Jane. *Herstory: A Womanifesto.* Self-published, 2015.

  - In *Herstory*, Jane recounts the ancient matriarchal societies, celebrating women's historical roles in nurturing and healing, and advocating for the resurgence of feminine power in modern life.

Supporting Works:

- **Baker, Jeannine Parvati.** *Prenatal Yoga & Natural Childbirth.* Self-published, 1986.

  - A foundational text that influenced Jane's approach to holistic birthing, this work focuses on natural childbirth and the wisdom of the female body.

- **World Health Organisation** (WHO). *Maternal and Newborn Health Policies.* Available at: https://www.who.int.

  - WHO guidelines advocate for respectful, supportive maternal care, aligning with Jane's focus on compassionate and empowering birthing practices.

Additional References:

- **Goldin, Claudia.** *The Quiet Revolution: The Pill's Impact on Women's Career and Family Decisions.* Harvard University Press, 2006.

  - This book provides an in-depth exploration of how the contraceptive pill affected women's roles in the workforce and family structures.

- **Bailey, Martha J.** *More Power to the Pill: The Impact of Contraceptive Freedom on Women's Life Cycle Labor Supply*. The Quarterly Journal of Economics, vol. 121, no. 1, 2006, pp. 289-320.

    o   This paper specifically addresses the effect of the pill on women's labor force participation, which connects to the reflection on the broader economic changes and dual-income households.

- **Grand View Research**. *Global Childcare Market Value to Reach $520 Billion by 2030*. Grand View Research, 2023.

    o   This report provides context for the discussion about the growth of the childcare industry as a result of changes in family structures driven by the rise of dual-income households.

- **LaingBuisson**. *UK Childcare Market Report 2020*. LaingBuisson, 2020.

    o   A key source for understanding how the need for childcare services increased in the UK following societal shifts in family and work dynamics.

- **Roberts, S. C., et al.** *Relationship Satisfaction and Outcome in Women Who Meet Their Partner While Using Oral Contraception*. Proceedings of the Royal Society B: Biological Sciences, vol. 279, no. 1732, 2012, pp. 1430-1436.

    o   This study explores how hormonal contraception impacts attraction and relationship satisfaction, supporting reflections on partner choice dynamics.

- **Guttmacher Institute.** *Contraceptive Use in the United States*. Guttmacher Institute, 2022.

    o   Provides updated data on contraceptive use, trends, and implications, framing the discussion on the pill's long-term influence on personal health and societal expectations.

- **Hillard, P. J. A.** *Menstrual Suppression: Current Perspectives.* International Journal of Women's Health, vol. 6, 2014, pp. 631-637.

  - This paper provides insight into the medical and psychological effects of menstrual suppression, which supports discussions on how the pill can alter women's natural cycles and intuition.

- **Pope, Alexandra, and Sjanie Hugo Wurlitzer.** *Wild Power: Discover the Magic of Your Menstrual Cycle and Awaken the Feminine Path to Power.* Hay House, 2017.

  - This book highlights the spiritual and personal growth potential of menstrual cycle awareness, aligning with Jane's advocacy for reconnecting with feminine power.

- **Red School.** *Menstrual Cycle Awareness: Harnessing the Power of Your Cycle for Growth and Well-being.* Available at: https://www.redschool.net.

  - Explores the importance of understanding and working with the menstrual cycle for personal development and well-being.

Chapter 5 - Dr. Christiane Northrup

Glossary of Terms

Menopause
The natural end of a woman's reproductive cycle, marking the cessation of menstruation and the transition into a new life phase. Dr. Northrup frames menopause as a time for self-discovery, empowerment, and personal growth.

The Mother of All Wake-Up Calls
Dr. Northrup's term for menopause as a profound call to self-awareness and authenticity. She describes it as a transformative period that urges women to reconnect with their true selves and embrace their life's purpose.

Perimenopause
The years leading up to menopause, characterised by hormonal fluctuations that can bring about physical and emotional changes. Dr. Northrup suggests viewing perimenopause as a preparatory phase, an opportunity to tune into one's body and prepare for the transition ahead.

Feminine Wisdom
Dr. Northrup's term for the intuitive understanding women have of their bodies and emotions, which grows stronger through life experiences such as menstruation, childbirth, and menopause.

Hormesis
A practice that involves exposing the body to mild, controlled stressors (such as exercise or intermittent fasting) to build resilience. Dr. Northrup advocates hormesis as a valuable approach to maintaining health and vitality as we age.

Goddesses Never Age
Dr. Northrup's philosophy is that aging should be embraced as a journey of joy, vitality, and empowerment rather than a process of decline. She encourages women to view aging as a time for self-renewal and inner strength.

Mind-Body Connection
The relationship between mental, emotional, and physical health. Dr. Northrup highlights the impact of thoughts and emotions on physical well-being, especially during menopause.

Medical Freedom
The principle of having autonomy and choice in healthcare decisions. Dr. Northrup supports medical freedom, encouraging individuals to make informed decisions aligned with their values and intuition.

Energy Vampires
A term Dr. Northrup uses to describe people who drain others' energy through negative or manipulative behaviours. She advises setting boundaries with such individuals to protect one's emotional and physical well-being.

Vital Life Force
The intrinsic energy that sustains health and vitality. According to Dr. Northrup, menopause is a time to renew this life force by focusing on joy, purpose, and connection with oneself.

Adrenal Fatigue
A condition caused by prolonged stress that depletes adrenal gland function, resulting in fatigue and burnout. Dr. Northrup emphasises the importance of adrenal health, especially during menopause, to manage stress effectively.

Female Hormones
The key hormones influencing a woman's reproductive cycle, including oestrogen, progesterone, testosterone, follicle-stimulating hormone (FSH), and luteinising hormone (LH). Dr. Northrup discusses how these hormones fluctuate during perimenopause and menopause, affecting physical and emotional well-being:

- **Oestrogen**: Crucial for reproductive health; its decline during menopause can lead to symptoms like hot flushes, mood swings, and changes in skin elasticity.

- **Progesterone**: Regulates the menstrual cycle and supports pregnancy. Declining levels may cause anxiety, irritability, and sleep disturbances during menopause.

- **Testosterone**: Influences libido, energy levels, and muscle mass. Declining levels during menopause can impact vitality and sexual well-being.

- **Follicle-Stimulating Hormone (FSH)**: Stimulates the growth of ovarian follicles; its rising levels during menopause indicate the transition is underway.

- **Luteinising Hormone (LH)**: Works with FSH to regulate the menstrual cycle; LH levels also increase as ovarian function declines.

Phytoestrogens
Plant-based compounds, found in foods like soy and flaxseed, that mimic oestrogen's effects in the body. Dr. Northrup

recommends phytoestrogens as a natural option for
supporting hormonal balance during menopause.

Bioidentical Hormones
Hormones that are chemically identical to those produced by
the human body. Dr. Northrup suggests bioidentical hormone
replacement therapy as a gentler option for managing
menopausal symptoms.

Chronic Inflammation
A prolonged inflammatory response that Dr. Northrup links to
ageing and various health issues. She promotes an anti-
inflammatory diet and lifestyle to manage inflammation,
especially during menopause.

Autophagy
The body's natural process of cellular cleansing and repair,
stimulated by practices like intermittent fasting. Dr. Northrup
recommends autophagy as a way to support healthy ageing.

Kundalini Energy
A concept describing latent energy believed to reside at the
base of the spine. Dr. Northrup sometimes references
Kundalini energy as part of the spiritual awakening that can
occur during menopause.

Oxytocin
Known as the 'love hormone,' oxytocin promotes bonding,
connection, and emotional well-being. Dr. Northrup
highlights its positive effects on mood and relationships,
particularly during life transitions.

Epigenetics
The study of how lifestyle factors influence gene expression.
Dr. Northrup suggests that women use menopause as an
opportunity to make lifestyle choices that positively affect
their health and well-being.

Law of Attraction
The belief that positive or negative thoughts bring
corresponding experiences into one's life. Dr. Northrup
incorporates the Law of Attraction into her teachings,

emphasising how mindset influences health, happiness, and quality of life.

References

Books by Dr. Christiane Northrup:

- **Northrup, Christiane.** *The Wisdom of Menopause: Creating Physical and Emotional Health During the Change.* New York: Bantam, 2020. ISBN-13: 978-0553386721.

    o   This foundational text provides guidance on navigating menopause as a powerful life transition, with practices that support holistic well-being.

- **Northrup, Christiane.** *Goddesses Never Age: The Secret Prescription for Radiance, Vitality, and Well-Being.* New York: Hay House, 2015. ISBN-13: 978-1401945954.

    o   Dr. Northrup redefines ageing as an empowering journey, encouraging women to embrace vitality and inner strength.

Supporting Works:

- **Martinez, Mario.** *The MindBody Code: How to Change the Beliefs that Limit Your Health, Longevity, and Success.* Boulder: Sounds True, 2014. ISBN-13: 978-1622032313.

    o   This book supports Dr. Northrup's emphasis on the mind-body connection, exploring how beliefs and thought patterns affect physical health and ageing.

Articles and Reports:

- **World Health Organisation** (WHO). *Health Guidelines for Aging.* Available at: https://www.who.int.

- o Global guidelines focused on maintaining wellness and quality of life as we age, aligning with Dr. Northrup's holistic approach to menopause.

Awards:

- **Zelenko Foundation**. Rosa Parks Fearless Stand for Medical Freedom Award (2022).

  - o Dr. Northrup received this award in recognition of her commitment to advocating autonomy and choice in healthcare.

Global Market Research:

Weight Loss Market:

- **Market Research Future.** *Global Weight Loss Market Size*. (2024). Retrieved from MRFR.

- **Statista.** *U.S. Weight Loss Market Value*. (2024). Retrieved from Statista.

- **Daxue Consulting**. *China's Weight Loss Market*. (2023). Retrieved from Daxue Consulting.

- **Nikkei Asia**. *Japan Weight Loss Market*. (2023). Retrieved from Nikkei Asia.

- **Statista**. *Germany Weight Loss Market*. (2023). Retrieved from Statista.

- **Euromonitor International.** *Brazil Weight Loss Market*. (2023). Retrieved from Euromonitor.

- **Mintel.** *UK Weight Loss Market*. (2023). Retrieved from Mintel.

- **BusinessWire**. *France Weight Loss Market*. (2023). Retrieved from BusinessWire.

- **IBISWorld.** *Australia Weight Loss Market*. (2023). Retrieved from IBISWorld.

Beauty Industry:

- **Statista.** *Global Beauty Industry Market Size.* (2024). Retrieved from Statista.

- **Grand View Research.** *Anti-Aging Market Projections.* (2024). Retrieved from Grand View Research.

- **Statista**. *U.S. Beauty Market Value.* (2024). Retrieved from Statista.

- **China Daily.** *China's Beauty Market.* (2023). Retrieved from China Daily.

- **CosmeticsDesign-Asia.** *Japan Beauty Market.* (2023). Retrieved from CosmeticsDesign-Asia.

- **Euromonitor International.** *Brazil Beauty Market.* (2023). Retrieved from Euromonitor.

- **Germany Trade & Invest (GTAI).** *Germany Beauty Market.* (2023). Retrieved from GTAI.

- **Korea Trade-Investment Promotion Agency** (KOTRA). *South Korea Beauty Market.* (2023). Retrieved from KOTRA.

- **India Brand Equity Foundation** (IBEF). *India Beauty Market Growth.* (2023). Retrieved from IBEF.

- **Business of Fashion**. *France Beauty Market.* (2023). Retrieved from BoF.

- **Mintel**. *UK Beauty Market.* (2023). Retrieved from Mintel.

- **Export.gov**. *Italy Beauty Market.* (2023). Retrieved from Export.gov.

Historical References on Menopause:

- **Wilson, R. A.** *Feminine Forever.* M. Evans & Company, 1966.

- **Utian, W. H.** *The True Therapeutic Rationale for the Use of Postmenopausal Estrogen Therapy.* American Journal of Obstetrics and Gynecology, 122(4), 370–375, 1975.

- **Rossouw, J. E., Anderson, G. L., Prentice, R. L., et al.** *Risks and Benefits of Estrogen Plus Progestin in Healthy Postmenopausal Women: Principal Results from the Women's Health Initiative Randomized Controlled Trial.* JAMA, 288(3), 321–333, 2002.

Chapter 6 - Dr. Vandana Shiva

Glossary of Terms

Seed Sovereignty
The right of farmers to save, share, and cultivate their own seeds without dependence on corporate-controlled patents. Dr. Shiva advocates for seed sovereignty as essential to preserving biodiversity, protecting farmers' rights, and ensuring food security in the face of corporate control.

Navdanya
An organisation founded by Dr. Shiva focused on promoting biodiversity, supporting organic farming, and establishing community seed banks. Navdanya has created over 150 seed banks across India and advocates for farmers' rights to sustainable, local agriculture.

Genetically Modified Organisms (GMOs)
Organisms whose DNA has been engineered to display traits such as pest resistance or higher yield. Dr. Shiva argues that GMOs harm biodiversity, degrade soil health, and create dependency on agrochemical corporations. She warns that GMOs, like Bt cotton, have led to pest resistance and increased chemical usage, ultimately damaging ecosystems and local farming traditions.

Bt Toxin
A toxin derived from the bacterium *Bacillus thuringiensis* (Bt) and engineered into crops like Bt cotton to kill pests. Dr. Shiva

highlights how pests are developing resistance to Bt crops, leading to increased pesticide use, greater environmental harm, and compromised biodiversity.

Roundup-Ready Crops
Genetically modified crops engineered to withstand glyphosate, the active ingredient in the herbicide Roundup. Dr. Shiva critiques Roundup-Ready crops for promoting excessive use of glyphosate, which has been linked to health and environmental risks. Overuse has led to 'superweeds' resistant to glyphosate, requiring even more intensive chemical applications and contributing to soil degradation.

The Great Reset
An economic recovery initiative proposed by the World Economic Forum in response to the COVID-19 pandemic. Dr. Shiva warns that the Great Reset, while claiming to promote sustainability, centralises power with corporations, undermining local autonomy and food sovereignty.

Ecofeminism
A movement connecting environmentalism with women's rights, emphasising women's traditional role in nurturing the Earth. Dr. Shiva's ecofeminist approach links the exploitation of nature with the marginalisation of women, calling for a collaborative, holistic approach to environmental stewardship.

Earth Democracy
A concept developed by Dr. Shiva advocating for justice, sustainability, and peace through local, community-led control over resources. In her book *Earth Democracy*, she calls for resistance to corporate globalisation in favour of preserving local ecosystems, cultures, and community-based food systems.

Soil Health
The vitality and fertility of soil, crucial for sustainable farming and food security. Dr. Shiva promotes practices like crop rotation and organic fertilisers to maintain soil health, warning that chemical-intensive farming depletes soil biodiversity and reduces agricultural resilience.

Food Sovereignty
The right of communities to define and control their own food systems, prioritising sustainable and local production over corporate-driven practices. Dr. Shiva sees food sovereignty as a foundation for resilient, self-reliant communities, less vulnerable to global market disruptions.

Monoculture
The agricultural practice of growing a single crop over large areas, often leading to soil degradation and vulnerability to pests. Dr. Shiva critiques monoculture for reducing biodiversity and weakening ecosystems, advocating for diverse farming practices that promote resilience.

Biodiversity
The variety of life within an ecosystem, which supports natural resilience and adaptability. Dr. Shiva argues that biodiversity is fundamental to sustainable agriculture and warns against practices that reduce it, such as monoculture farming and the use of GMOs.

Colonialism in Agriculture
Dr. Shiva describes modern industrial agriculture as a form of 'colonialism,' where corporations impose control over farmers and local resources, disrupting traditional practices and creating dependency. She argues that this corporate model perpetuates inequality and threatens food sovereignty.

Fourth Industrial Revolution
The convergence of digital, physical, and biological technologies, including AI and robotics. Dr. Shiva is concerned that this shift centralises power in the hands of corporations, particularly in agriculture, undermining traditional farming practices and local autonomy.

Quantum Theory and Interconnectedness
Drawing on her background in physics, Dr. Shiva uses the concept of interconnectedness in quantum theory as a metaphor for the interdependence of life on Earth. This principle underpins her ecofeminist beliefs and her commitment to holistic environmental activism.

The Commons
Resources such as land, water, and air that are shared by everyone and are essential for life. Dr. Shiva advocates for the protection of these commons, arguing that they should remain public resources and not be privatised by corporations.

References

Books by Dr. Vandana Shiva:

- **Shiva, Vandana**. *Earth Democracy: Justice, Sustainability, and Peace*. Cambridge, MA: South End Press, 2005. ISBN-13: 978-0896087450.

- **Shiva, Vandana**. *Stolen Harvest: The Hijacking of the Global Food Supply*. Cambridge, MA: South End Press, 2000. ISBN-13: 978-0896086071.

- **Shiva, Vandana, and Kartikey Shiva**. *Oneness vs. the 1%: Shattering Illusions, Seeding Freedom*. New Delhi: Women Unlimited, 2020. ISBN-13: 978-1944835002.

Articles and Reports:

- **World Economic Forum.** *The Great Reset*. Published 2020. Available at: https://www.weforum.org/great-reset.

- **International Monetary Fund**. *The Impact of Colonialism on Global Development*. Available at: https://www.imf.org.

- **Vanguard Group and BlackRock Inc.** Financial Reports. Available at: https://www.blackrock.com and https://www.vanguard.com.

Public Speeches and Lectures:

- Key speeches at the United Nations and global forums advocating for biodiversity, food sovereignty, and ecofeminism.

- TEDx talks and documentaries such as *The World According to Monsanto*, which feature her critiques of industrial agriculture and GMOs.

Organisational References:

- **Navdanya:** Foundational papers and reports from Navdanya, the organisation founded by Dr. Shiva, advocating for seed sovereignty and the conservation of biodiversity.

- Global campaigns like the Seed Freedom movement, which highlight the importance of preserving indigenous agricultural practices.

Scientific Studies and Collaborative Research:

- Peer-reviewed studies critiquing the Green Revolution's environmental and social impacts.

- Research collaborations between ecologists, agronomists, and Navdanya on sustainable agricultural practices.

Cultural and Spiritual Connections:

- References to the Indian philosophical concept of *Vasudhaiva Kutumbakam* ('The world is one family'), which underpins her ecofeminist worldview.

- Indigenous farming and seed-saving traditions that align with her advocacy for sustainability and biodiversity.

Media Coverage and Documentaries:

- Documentaries like *The World According to Monsanto* delve into industrial agriculture's consequences and feature Shiva's work.

- Investigative news reports and interviews covering her campaigns and activism.

Legislative and Policy Reports:

- The Cartagena Protocol on Biosafety and its implications for biodiversity protection.

- Policies addressing GMOs and environmental sustainability, aligning with Shiva's advocacy.

Reflection-Specific References:

- Dr. Shiva's metaphors of seeds as symbols of regeneration, resilience, and life cycles, drawn from her writings and speeches.

- Connections between personal growth, life transitions, and the cycles of nature, echoing Shiva's ecofeminist philosophy.

Appendix: 1 Navigating Menopause Together A Partner's Guide

References

1. **Northrup, C.** (2012). *The Wisdom of Menopause.* Bantam.

2. **Weed, S. S.** (2002). *New Menopausal Years the Wise Woman Way.* Ash Tree Publishing.

3. **Kabat-Zinn, J.** (1990). *Full Catastrophe Living.* Delacorte.

4. **Estés, C. P.** (1992). *Women Who Run With the Wolves.* Ballantine Books.

5. **Siegel, B. S.** (1986). *Love, Medicine, and Miracles.* Harper & Row.

6. **Mayo Clinic.** (n.d.). *Menopause: Symptoms and Causes.* Retrieved from www.mayoclinic.org.

7. **McGarey, G.** (2023). *A Well-Lived Life.* Atria Books.

Appendix 2 - Empower Your Care
Key Questions to Ask Your Doctor During
Menopause

References

1. **Weed, S. S.** (2002). *New Menopausal Years the Wise Woman Way*. Ash Tree Publishing.

2. **Mayo Clinic.** (n.d.). *Menopause: Hormone Therapy*. Retrieved from www.mayoclinic.org.

3. **McGarey, G.** (2023). *A Well-Lived Life: A 102-Year-Old Doctor's Six Secrets to Health and Happiness at Every Age*. Atria Books.

4. **North American Menopause Society (NAMS).** (n.d.). *Clinical Practice Guidelines for Menopause Management*. Retrieved from www.menopause.org.

5. **Northrup, C.** (2012). *The Wisdom of Menopause*. Bantam.

6. **Siegel, B. S.** (1986). *Love, Medicine, and Miracles*. Harper & Row.

7. **Kabat-Zinn, J.** (1990). *Full Catastrophe Living*. Delacorte.

8. **Pope, A., & Wurlitzer, S.** (2017). *Wild Power*. Hay House.

Appendix: 3 Menopause Symptoms and Their Spiritual Messages

References

1. **Northrup, C.** (2012). *The Wisdom of Menopause*. Bantam.

2. **Weed, S. S.** (2002). *New Menopausal Years the Wise Woman Way*. Ash Tree Publishing.

3. **Pope, A., & Wurlitzer, S.** (2017). *Wild Power*. Hay House.

4. **Kabat-Zinn, J.** (1990). *Full Catastrophe Living*. Delacorte.

5. **Estés, C. P.** (1992). *Women Who Run With the Wolves*. Ballantine Books.

6. **Siegel, B. S.** (1986). *Love, Medicine, and Miracles*. Harper & Row.

7. **McGarey, G.** (2023). *A Well-Lived Life*. Atria Books.

8. **Mayo Clinic**. (n.d.). *Menopause: Symptoms and Causes*. Retrieved from www.mayoclinic.org.

Disclaimer

(Governed by Australian Law, Common Law, and Global Humanitarian Law)

This book, The Seven Wonders of Menopause, is provided for informational and educational purposes only. It reflects the author's personal research, experiences, and interpretations, as well as voluntary contributions from individuals featured in its pages. It is not a substitute for professional medical, legal, financial, or other expert advice. Readers are strongly encouraged to consult qualified professionals and conduct independent research before making decisions based on the content of this book.

Dynamic Nature of Information

The information contained in this book was accurate to the best of the author's knowledge at the time of writing. However, ongoing developments may render some information outdated, incomplete, or inaccurate. The author and publisher assume no obligation to update or revise the content after publication. Readers are responsible for verifying the relevance of the information to their circumstances.

Consent and Permissions from Contributors

All individuals featured in this book have voluntarily shared their stories, fully aware of their inclusion in this publication. Contributors have reviewed and approved the final presentation of their contributions, and all necessary permissions have been obtained. The author and publisher are not responsible for any changes in contributors' personal views, circumstances, or experiences after publication.

Privacy and Confidentiality Waiver

All contributors have provided informed consent for the publication of their stories. The author and publisher disclaim liability for any emotional, financial, or reputational consequences experienced by contributors as a result of their participation.

Limitation of Liability and Assumption of Risk

In accordance with Section 64A of the Australian Consumer Law (Competition and Consumer Act 2010) and the Volenti non fit injuria (common law principle), readers acknowledge that any actions taken based on this book's content are at their own risk. The author and publisher are not liable for any loss, injury, harm, or damages—direct, indirect, incidental, or consequential—resulting from the use or misuse of the information provided.

No Endorsements or Recommendations

References to specific companies, products, services, or individuals are for illustrative purposes only and do not constitute endorsements or recommendations. Readers are advised to conduct their own research before engaging with any referenced entities.

Copyright, Fair Use, and Intellectual Property

This book may reference third-party material under the fair use provisions of the Copyright Act 1968 (Cth). These materials are included for educational, commentary, or critical purposes. The author and publisher assert no proprietary rights over third-party content. If copyrighted material has been inadvertently included without proper attribution, corrections or removals will be made upon notification.

No Defamation or Malice

This book was written in good faith and reflects the author's opinions. It is intended to educate, inspire, and engage in critical discussion. In accordance with the Defamation Act 2005 (Vic), the author disclaims any intent to defame, harm, or malign any individual, company, or organisation. Any resemblance to real events, persons, or entities is purely coincidental unless explicitly stated.

Jurisdiction and Governing Law

This disclaimer and any legal disputes arising from this book are governed by the laws of Victoria, Australia, under the Judiciary Act 1903 (Cth) and the Conflict of Laws (Foreign Elements) Act 1993 (Vic). All legal claims must be filed exclusively in the courts of Victoria, Australia. By reading, purchasing, or using this book, you agree to submit to the jurisdiction of these courts, regardless of your location.

Global Applicability and Reader Consent

This disclaimer applies worldwide. By purchasing or reading this book, you consent to the terms outlined herein and acknowledge that all legal matters must be resolved under Australian law in Victoria's courts. Legal action in other jurisdictions is not permitted against the author or publisher.

Digital and Online Content

If this book is distributed digitally, the author and publisher are not responsible for misuse, unauthorised distribution, or alterations made to its content in digital formats. Readers are advised to verify the authenticity of any digital copies through official sources.

Final Waiver of Liability

By continuing to read or use this book, you release the author and publisher from any liability for harm, loss, or damages—whether physical, emotional, or financial—arising from the use or interpretation of the content. The reader assumes full responsibility for all decisions and actions taken based on this book. Outcomes resulting from outdated information, misinterpretation, or unauthorised third-party use are not the responsibility of the author or publisher.

About the Author

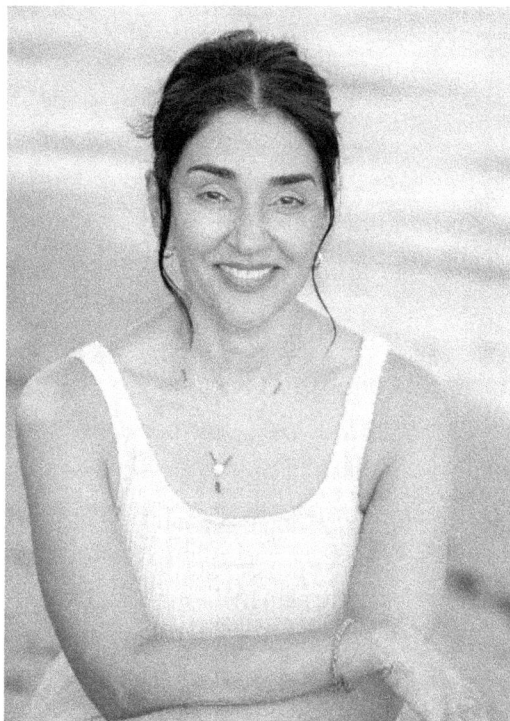

Shavita Kotak

Photo credit: Ruth Schwarzenholz

Like many of you, I've spent my life moving through different roles and experiences, each one shaping the woman I am today. I was born in London to Indian parents, navigating the tensions between cultural expectations and self-discovery. Over the years, life has taken me on a wild ride—from working as a financial planner in Australia to becoming a mother and finally embracing my true calling as a seeker of knowledge and wisdom. I understand the challenges and joys that come with these roles, and I hope my experiences can offer you comfort and guidance.

My journey through perimenopause and motherhood was anything but smooth—it was confusing, messy, and, at times, overwhelming. But in those challenges, I found something unexpected: a deeper connection to myself, a spiritual awakening that redefined how I see life. I realised that menopause isn't an end; it's a powerful beginning—a chance to let go of old expectations and step fully into who we are meant to be.

This book, *The Seven Wonders of Menopause*, was born from nearly a decade of research, reflection, and personal transformation. It's a collection of wisdom, stories, and conversations with remarkable women who have inspired me along the way—Dr. Gladys McGarey, a healer and pioneer who showed us the power of living with purpose at any age; Robin Lim, who taught me about the sacred connection between birth, life, and spirit; Jane Hardwicke Collings, whose work with rites of passage deepened my understanding of transitions; Alexandra Pope, a visionary who opened my eyes to the wisdom within the menstrual cycle; Dr. Christiane Northrup, whose teachings gave me strength to navigate menopause as a spiritual journey; and Dr. Vandana Shiva, who reminded me that healing the earth and healing ourselves are deeply intertwined.

Each of these women helped shape the path I walk today. Their voices and my own are woven throughout this book to offer a glimpse of what's possible when we embrace change, reclaim our power, and live from a place of truth.

Life is not a straight line—it's a series of cycles. Each stage invites us to reflect, release, and reinvent ourselves. Through this book, I hope to inspire other women to see menopause not as something to fear but as an opportunity to step into their truth and claim the power that comes with age.

When I'm not writing or facilitating women's circles, I spend time with my family, practice yoga, travel to sacred places, or enjoy life's little joys—good music, deep conversations, and moments of stillness.

This journey isn't just mine—it belongs to all of us. Together, we rise, embrace change, and discover that the best is yet to come.

Connect with Shavita Kotak

For more information about Shavita's offerings, events, and workshops, visit her website at shivitakotak.com. You can also follow her on social media, where she shares her insights and wisdom about the spiritual journey of menopause and beyond. Shavita inspires others to embrace transformation with courage, grace, and intention through her work.

www.ingramcontent.com/pod-product-compliance
Lightning Source LLC
Chambersburg PA
CBHW031116020426
42333CB00012B/107